The Shape of the Eye

Advance Praise for *The Shape of the Eye*

"A poignant, beautifully written, and intensely moving memoir. I think only one writer in the world, George Estreich, could possibly have pulled this off. It will become part of the canon of narratives that are studied and taught in medical humanities courses."

—**Abraham Verghese**, author of *Cutting for Stone*

"This is the story of Laura, a girl with Down syndrome who taught a family to love with ordinary perfection and uncommon relevance. Expect to be taken on a journey, too, as Laura asks: What's most important in your life?"

—**Brian Skotko**, MD, MPP, co-author of
Common Threads: Celebrating Life with Down Syndrome

"*The Shape of the Eye* is a story of misunderstanding, devastating pain, and overwhelming challenge. It is also a story of intense bonds between a man and a woman, between parent and child, and between family and community. It is a story of growth and learning. Ultimately it is a story, beautifully written, of loyalty, affection, persistence, and the most important human victory, which is love."

—**Robert Morgan**, author of *Gap Creek*

"A story that refuses to sentimentalize, that takes a hard look at Down syndrome and our culture's response to it. At heart, *The Shape of the Eye* is the story of a little girl and her family. Told with wit, warmth, and honesty, it's ultimately a human story of a lucky life."

—**Lee Martin**, author of *The Bright Forever*

"A rich, compelling, and instructive memoir, potentially illuminating and helpful both to persons raising children with special needs—and Down syndrome especially—and to those families' professional health care providers. The book is interesting and valuable as an informative, sensitive exploration of the growing phenomenon of American fathers staying home to be the primary caretakers for their children. Estreich's candor about his experience, the ensuing family dynamics, and the myriad social implications of this role is impressive. A valuable contribution."

—**Marcia Day Childress**,
director of the Programs in Humanities,
University of Virginia School of Medicine

Medical Humanities

Thomas Mayo, series editor

The Shape of the Eye

Down Syndrome, Family, and the Stories We Inherit

George Estreich

Afterword by Marcia Day Childress

Southern Methodist University Press / Dallas

Requests for permission to reproduce material from this work should be sent to:
Rights and Permissions
Southern Methodist University Press
PO Box 750415
Dallas, Texas 75275-0415

Cover photo: Laura at age seven by George Estreich
Jacket and text design by Kellye Sanford

Library of Congress Cataloging-in-Publication Data

Estreich, George.
The shape of the eye : Down syndrome, family, and the stories we inherit / George
Estreich ; afterword by Marcia Day Childress. — 1st ed.
p. cm. — (Medical humanities)
Includes bibliographical references.
Summary: Writer George Estreich describes how raising a child with Down syndrome
impacted everything else in his life, including his approach to writing
and the way he now perceives other events in his own life and in the lives of his
family members.
ISBN 978-0-87074-567-6 (alk. paper)
1. Estreich, Laura Regina. 2. Down syndrome—Patients—Biography. 3. Down syndrome—
Patients—Family relationships. 4. Children with disabilities—Biography.
5. Estreich, George. 6. Estreich, George—Family. 7. Parents of children with disabilities—
Biography. 8. Authors, American—Biography. 9. Stay at home fathers—Biography. I. Title.
II. Series: Medical humanities.
RJ506.D68E88 2011
618.92'85884200922—dc22

2010043450

Printed in the United States of America on acid-free paper

10   9   8   7   6   5   4   3

for Ellie

Contents

Introduction

We were waiting for our family doctor. I felt—not serene, but expectant. Uncertain. Theresa lifted Laura from her car seat and set her, still sleeping, on the clean white paper of the exam table. I got out colored pencils and a notebook for Ellie. We were paging through magazines when Dr. E. came in, knocking softly. He closed the door, crossed the room, and turned towards us.

"We got the lab tests back," he said. "Nancy called and had them faxed down here." He paused.

"Laura does have Down syndrome," he said.

Ellie was coloring quietly. From where I was standing, I could see the first tears forming in Theresa's eyes.

"I believe," he said, "that these children come to the families most able to take care of them."

No one said anything. Ellie kept drawing her rainbow, keeping the colored lines parallel. There was a bump in the first line she'd drawn, and she copied it through all the succeeding lines, the blip softening into a gentle swell. Ellie, meticulous, precise, absorbed. She didn't seem to register the news. Theresa stared up at the doctor, her eyes wet. I felt nothing, only the grip of fact, so I began asking questions, setting them out like planks heaved across quicksand. What do we do. Whom do we contact. What do we need to know.

I thought a lot about that moment in the weeks following. The way Dr. E. turned towards us, the door easing towards an institutional click. His face, pinker than usual, the hush in his voice, his gentleness. All said that the news was coming. Laura did have Down syndrome. The question attending her birth had been answered, but that answer only seemed another question. Or it was, like the chromosome itself, the beginning of a thousand questions. Clearly an answer was called for.

I began to read. I wanted to understand what Laura had.

Down syndrome, as I learned, is a chromosomal disorder. Chromosomes are long strings of DNA, the molecule that encodes inheritance; taken together, they constitute a genome, a full set of instructions for guiding development from the fertilized egg. Most people have forty-six chromosomes: twenty-three from Mom, twenty-three from Dad, a perfectly matched set. People with the main form of Down syndrome have an extra copy of the twenty-first chromosome, the smallest. Because that extra copy is present at conception, it is preserved faithfully through each successive cell division, and ten trillion cells or so later, it is ubiquitous in the body.

Having an extra chromosome makes for significant changes. People with Down syndrome have a distinctive look, almost always with almond-shaped eyes; they have some degree of intellectual disability, usually in the mild to moderate range; and they're at increased risk for a number of medical problems, including heart defects, intestinal malformations, and leukemia, though an individual child may have none of these. There are also features you wouldn't notice if you weren't looking for them, like a single line across the palm.

Writing this description, I know it is necessary and misleading, accurate and deeply false. A *syndrome* means, at root, a "running together." When you have a child, it all runs together: the heart defect, the eyes, the way her voice sounds, the name of the speech therapist, the worries over the future, the joys of discovery, the sliding sense—slow, quiet, enormous, an avalanche in the skull—that *different* is not as different as you thought. The genes produce the child, who lives a story, whose story is bound up with yours. So reducing a child to a heap of medical fragments is, for a parent, a complicated and dissonant act. It is a necessary fiction, a story one tells only in order to move on.

Nobody, so far as I know, finds out that a newborn child has Down syndrome, shrugs, and returns to decorating the nursery. We were undone by the news for a long time. If Down syndrome were ordinary in the world, if a commonsense view of dignity and personhood and capability prevailed, then perhaps our early days would have been easier. But Down syndrome is not ordinary in the world.

I kept looking things up. Against whispers in my own brain, against shocked silence, against the raw unfamiliarity of our newest family member, I turned to fact. I felt not just ignorant, but *culpably* ignorant. And yet in my reading, I only found my own confusion writ large.

I felt that Laura's life was valuable, that she was a child, a sister and daughter and granddaughter above all, that she might learn and thrive. I also felt that our lives were over, that her birth was a tragedy, and that we were condemned to a half-life of hospitals, acronyms, therapists, and forms. In my unhinged research, I discovered that everything was true. She was "a child first"—but of course, she could have this problem, and this one, and this one, and this one. Or the big list came first, typically framed as *they*: they have heart defects, intestinal atresias, low IQs, joint problems, and on and on. Oh, but they are happy little tykes! None of it made sense. I did not see how a child could be happy if she had so many problems; I did not see how, with so many problems, she could be "a child first." I had sought refuge in fact, like someone who ducks into a cathedral for quiet, and instead finds an echo chamber for every footfall. Or I *was* the echo chamber, thronged with a dense collision of numbers and hope and resignation.

There were, it seemed, two kinds of stories told about my daughter. In one, she seemed to be a developing child. In the other, she seemed not even human. She was a defect, a tragedy, an abnormality. I did not see how she could be both. It was as if Theresa had given birth to a blur.

The Shape of the Eye

Arrival

Laura was born at 7:02 on a late February morning, after a labor Theresa described as "blessedly brief." I woke up around three, hearing Theresa say, "George. I think my water just broke." "Okay," I said, "okay okay okay." I began stuffing underwear and socks into an overnight bag. We called Kai, who came over to stay with Ellie. We woke up Ellie and told her we were going to the hospital. She mumbled something and went back to sleep. The first and second contractions were eleven minutes apart. Theresa wanted to strip the bed. She wanted to *red up* a little, the Pittsburgh slang for tidying. The second and third contractions were four minutes apart. I objected to the *redding up*. We hurried out to the Subaru. Four hours later, Laura was born, without anesthesia or complications, in a half-empty maternity ward. She weighed seven pounds, three and a half ounces.

We were allowed a few hours of ignorance. Our nameless daughter was whisked off for the obligatory bath, eyedrops, and heel stick. She was gone for a long time, but I didn't suspect a thing.

Later that day, Dr. E. came to see us in the hospital. Ever since we'd moved to Oregon, Kevin Ewanchyna—Dr. E., to most—had helped Ellie through the colds, ear infections, and vaccinations of an ordinary childhood. Sandy-haired and neat, circumspect, a trace of Canada in his vowels, he'd arrived in Corvallis at about the same time we did, and we'd lucked into his practice. He congratulated us, greeted Ellie warmly, and began to examine Baby Girl Estreich. As he moved the stethoscope's disk lightly across her chest, he seemed more intent than usual. When he mentioned Down syndrome, a silence sharpened in the room, but the moment passed.

It was the first hint of what was already true, and you would think Dr. E.'s words would be seared in memory. And yet, even though I have memorized many of my friends' license plates and can recite the supporting actors for movies I have not even seen, I cannot recall exactly how Dr. E. broke the news. Perhaps the possibility was too out of place to process, like a living image in an animated world. Perhaps it seemed too unlikely to dwell on, or too dire. As Dr. E. hastened to point out, many typical features were absent. There was no heart murmur. The palate was not cleft; it was not even highly arched, though the arch was somewhat pronounced. The "simian crease," a single line across the palm, was absent. And though most babies with Down syndrome are hypotonic—"floppy"—our daughter's muscle tone seemed good. What defied explanation were her eyes. They were vaguely Asian, almond-shaped, the same striking appearance that had led to the condition's original name: *Mongolian idiocy*. Fortunately, I had the answer for that one. My mother is Japanese.

We consented to the test for Down syndrome. Somewhere in Portland, a pathologist would isolate a nucleus from one of Laura's cells. Then he would stain the chromosomes, count them under a microscope, and disclose the range of possible futures. It was, as Dr. E. said, "for peace of mind." He left the room. A little later, a nurse came in, drew blood, and said we would know in a week.

Balloons arrived, flowers, baskets of jellybeans. There were phone calls, e-mails. Through it all, Down syndrome was there and not there, a tremor, a disturbance, a mirage. It was the universe a half step to the left, one we might enter, might not enter, had already entered. It was there in a phrase like *simian crease*—I thought, isn't that kind of, well, offensive? It was in the long pause as another doctor cradled our daughter's head in beefy hands, intent, compassionate, saying, "I notice the eyes are slightly almond-shaped"; and it was in my quick, already-automatic response, saying, "My mother is Japanese." I held up one generation against another. I held up what I was, against what she might be.

Ellie waited patiently for us to quit talking. She was seething with happy uncertainty. She wanted nothing other than the chance to hold her sister, and to stay within six inches of Theresa at all times. The three of them snuggled in the bed. We asked her what she thought about her little sister. "Good," she said, with emphasis, drawing out the vowel, as she only did for the best things: sleepovers, cotton candy, new sibling. We asked her about names. "What about Esmerelda?" said Theresa. "*Mom*," said Ellie. I said, "What about Sillyhead?" "Dad," she said, "stop it." I said, "What if we call her Ellie Is a Sillyhead? That way we could say Ellie Is a Sillyhead every time we wanted to talk to her." "*Dad*," she said, reproving. Clearly the situation's gravity had escaped me.

It was the end of February in a dry winter. Normally, in western Oregon, the rain begins in October, and doesn't really end until July. But it had been sunny, and all winter we walked around guiltily enjoying the good weather, which we knew we'd pay for, down the road, in wildfires and reduced salmon runs. We didn't care. It was nice out and we weren't suffering from SAD. It felt like that in the hospital, a temporary stay, a grace period, the sunlight shedding calm possibility through plate glass. The next morning, as Theresa and our second daughter slept upstairs, I sat in the hospital cafeteria with Ellie, eating dry scrambled eggs and French toast. I glanced idly at the new wing under construction next door, its broad webwork of shadows falling across the completed building, the bundled rebar and coils of wire piled in future rooms. Back upstairs, men in hardhats were asking directions through the pleasant beiges and stenciled decorations of the maternity ward.

Baby Girl Estreich was *Laura* now. The day before, I'd driven home to get the paperback full of names. In the room, I'd thumbed through the pages, a tiny telephone book of future lives, and read out possibilities. Nothing seemed right until I said *Laura*. The name fit, in the way *Eleanor* had, for Ellie. Theresa wanted Laura's middle name to be *Regina*, after her father Regis; there was a symmetry, both grandfathers, both passed on, represented in a name. *Laura Regina Estreich*. We liked it, though we hadn't planned it. We'd been thinking of the short list left over from *Eleanor*, but it seemed better, somehow, to start over.

Named, plugged into the system, Laura was free to go. We signed the discharge papers. I slipped our copies into the plastic bag, next to the sheet inked with Laura's footprints. I slung the duffle over my shoulder, and the nurse checked our ID bracelets against Laura's, before wheeling us out. Strangers beamed at us in the elevator. The nurse inspected our infant car seat. She shooed the smokers away from the hospital entrance. We told her about the lab tests we were waiting on, and she said, "Yes, some of us were wondering about that."

By the time we returned for our two-week checkup, we had discounted the possibility of Down syndrome. Laura was nursing, if not with the avid concentration her older sister had shown, then well enough. She could track a set of jingled keys. I'd been thinking about the possibility, though, so I'd called Dr. E.'s office after a week had passed. Nancy, Dr. E.'s nurse, said they were still waiting on the lab, but sometimes these things took a little longer.

We could not go back. We could not undo the crucial moment, the precise and unrecorded time of day when the initial error in cell division occurred, adding an extra chromosome to the beginning of what Laura would be. Now the infant before us bore that chromosome in every cell. It was in the shape of her eyes, the texture of her hair, in her brain and joints and heart.

I wanted to rewind the tape to the day before, to a refrigerator filled with casseroles baked by neighbors and friends, phone calls from family back East, and Ellie eager to hold Laura: she sat crosslegged on the carpet, her arms stiffly ready. We lowered Laura towards her, saying, *careful, support her head*, remembering how fragile Ellie had seemed, five and a half years ago. A weak afternoon sunlight splayed its rhombus across them. Laura blinked. Her hands opened and closed slowly, with no force, and I dandled my index finger against the translucent fingertips, marveling at the improbable size of newborn children: they seem scaled to another world. I remembered feeling the same way with Ellie, and felt the pleasure of layered time, the easy spiral of repetition and variation, intricate as a Bach invention. I looked at Laura's eyes, thought of my mother, and was reassured. We smiled down at our infant.

For a long time, I remembered this ignorance with intense nostalgia. We were under a spell: we had wished for normalcy and been granted two weeks, a time outside time, when we could hope for anything at all. Since our wish was not denied, denial made it true. When the spell was broken, the child before us assumed her true appearance—or say, instead, that her identity was revealed, that the centrifuge performed its necessary separations, and that her appearance was revealed in turn. She was unchanged and transformed. The palate was definitely arched, though not extremely so. The heart murmur was faint, but there.

Theresa said she felt as if our baby had been stolen, and replaced with a collection of medical problems. Steadying her voice seemed a pure act of will: the sobs that racked her reminded me of the birth. I listened, blank, disoriented. Past and present had been disjoined; pattern, as I knew it, was gone; Laura was not like Ellie; the days after Ellie's birth were not like this. Theresa had wept then, as well, but her predominant mood was joy. A research scientist to the core, she would smile through tears and say, Hormone levels. I remembered the river of time widening, slowing, the current broadening almost to stillness, our vistas a plain of light. We'd had that again for two weeks, a bright sure forward-moving calm, and it had led to the lip of a waterfall.

We turned to research. What we learned did not console us. There was no ground to fact: the hard bright particular grains added up to quicksand, a dry drowning. Early intervention, one booklet explained, is the key to continued progress. Children with Down syndrome tend to have hypotonia, or low muscle tone. If you did not do the special neck-strengthening exercises their heads would loll. Until they gained head control they would not sit up. Until they could sit up they would not crawl, and so on. And muscles are required for speech, for control of the complex mouth-shapes required for language, shapes made more difficult by deformed palates and thickened tongues. We would need a speech pathologist to assess Laura's abilities and to prescribe exercises, like sucking Jell-O through a straw. These lessons, of course, depended on communication. Language acquisition, early language acquisition, was key to further mental development. Language depended on hearing, another problem area, likely as not. We should test hearing every six months. We might consider learning sign language. Contact your local social services agency, the booklet advised. They can help you get in touch with the specialists your child's development requires.

Then there were the medical problems. Laura's chances of having a cardiac defect were about one in two; for a serious defect, requiring surgery, the chances were one in four. There are gastrointestinal problems, ranging from constipation to an imperforate anus, the simple absence of a hole. There are immune deficiencies, flat feet, respiratory ailments, nearsightedness. There is an increased risk of leukemia.

It can be overwhelming, one pamphlet consoled. You will need time to grieve for the child you did not have, and to recover from the shock. It then continued: an echocardiogram should be performed, and a pediatric cardiologist should be consulted as soon as possible.

Two days after the diagnosis, we returned to the hospital for an ultrasound of Laura's heart. In outline, the experience was familiar—the darkened room, the blue smear of gel, the amplified *whish whish whish*—but it felt wrong, an ultrasound after the birth, and when I looked into the aqueous cone of light on the monitor, I recognized nothing. There was no proto-human shape, no sudden recognition of head and feet. I saw only movement, a soft changing architecture of muscle, the view flexing as the tech angled the sensor, this way and that, against Laura's chest. A flurry of key clicks, and a kind of fire appeared, superimposed on the heart, blue and orange pixels flickering in sync with Laura's pulse, the colors mixing. Then another click, and the fire vanished, then the heart, replaced by the sediment of a ghostly earth: ribbons, folds, broken gaps, the folded rock of geological time. What's that, we asked, and the tech said she would rather defer to the cardiologist.

Later that day we got the results. The exact diagnosis would be confirmed later by the pediatric cardiologist in Portland, but the preliminary results were clear. Laura had an atrioventricular canal defect, a problem found almost exclusively among children with Down syndrome. In essence, the heart had failed to complete its development: the valves were unfinished, the walls between leaked with three separate holes. There was mitral regurgitation, blood backwashing through a leaky valve. This was the murmur the doctor had heard; this was the fire I'd seen. Given the magnitude of the defect, Laura would probably need surgery. In the meantime we should try to keep her from getting upset.

If you had asked me, before my child was born, what I wanted her to be, I would have told you I didn't care: I wanted her to be healthy and happy. If she didn't want to go to college, well, that would be fine, and I would support whatever life choices she made. I was assuming, of course, that a person with forty-six chromosomes would be making these decisions. Now I wondered about everything I had taken for granted with Ellie, the assumptions undisturbed by the microscopic. I wondered if Laura would have friends. I wondered if she would go on dates, if I would need to chaperone. Though I believed she would not go to college, I discovered that I might one day be wrong: some people with Down syndrome do attend college. I wondered if she would have to live her whole life with us. (She may.) I wondered how long she would live. The future seemed at once unreal and massively heavy, as if we could feel the atmosphere's weight.

We had begun, hesitantly, to tell others. And the question, whether spoken or not, was always: Did you test? One mother, when Theresa answered that we had not, asked *why not*, in disbelief, almost in anger. Her implication was clear: this all could have been avoided. Theresa recounted it later, and both of us were righteous, furious, loyal to the child we did not know. And yet it was hard, sometimes, not to question the decision. Our lives had changed overnight; Laura's heart surgery was immediately ahead; beyond that was the siege war of inclusion. It was never Laura we regretted: she charmed us from the beginning. It was the new life we feared.

We'd decided against fetal testing. Since Theresa wouldn't have chosen an abortion, there was no reason to test; the triple screen, because of its high false positive rate, could at best indicate the need for amniocentesis, which carried a small but real risk of miscarriage. For my part, I'd said to Theresa, early in the second trimester, that we'd take whoever came out. Our choice—or the choice Theresa made, and I assented to—was applied self-knowledge, a hedge against regret. We knew that given who we were, an abortion would invite a durable grief into our lives.

Now that Laura was here, we felt something like the grief we had sought to avoid, and because we were grieving a phantom, our feelings betrayed the actual child before us. Each question had an aftertaste of guilt. Had we done the right thing? Should we have tested? Had we been selfish? Had we, wanting Ellie to have a sibling, saddled her with a burden? Had we really considered what it meant to raise a disabled child? Had we conveniently mistaken the unlikely for the impossible? Now, evidently, the possibility was considering us. The hypothetical had hair, hands that clenched and unclenched softly, eyes to look around. People said she looked like me.

I felt foolish, bemused. Like it or not, I had constructed a future, one nearly as specific and complete as Laura herself; and that future, that nine-month reverie, was completely, provably wrong. Even as the forty-seventh chromosome added itself to each cell and differentiating system, brain, eyes, hair, defect-perforated heart, I, too, had been forming a life. Or, more exactly, a paralife, a hazy projection of new child and altered family. I expected, I suppose, a boy—that seemed balanced, one boy, one girl. He would be the rebellious one. There would be arguments. I reminded myself not to compare the two children, and not to expect too much. I steeled myself for a busier life, for increased stress and reduced writing time. Parents with two kids would say, "The second child changes everything, you have no idea," and I would say, "I know, I know." Everyone agreed there was no way to imagine it until you got there.

A Child First

We met in 1983, near the end of our first year at the University of Virginia, in the Pleistocene era of what was not even a relationship but is now a marriage, when my hair was long and I still drank herbal tea. We were eighteen years old. We sat on the floor of Theresa's dorm room, talking, then silent. I didn't mind the silences. They felt fine. Besides, I was nursing a low-grade depression that I hoped was mysteriously attractive. Theresa furrowed her brow, pinwheeled a pencil through her fingers, looked unsure of what to say. I liked her right away—liked her liked her—but with one thing and another, other entanglements, the usual fears, the poet unable to communicate his feelings, we were just friends for a long time.

It's safe to say that neither of us was thinking about Down syndrome then. But it may be that Laura's story had already begun: that the nondisjunction had already occurred, and the extra twenty-first chromosome was already present, ready to shape a face, a heart, a child trailed by murmurs. If our lives were a tragedy we would call this fate, the thread of inheritance spun out of the dark of family, the ancient fault surfacing in a new ruin. But our lives are not tragic, only puzzling, most of the time.

It's all dead-end metaphysics anyway, irrelevant to daily life. Whether the extra chromosome was waiting for years to shape our lives, or whether it arrived later, like a mysterious guest stepping off a train, is simply unknowable; and if we *could* know it, that certainty would not console. *All* of our chromosomes reach backwards into the past, into a darkness we cannot see, so to tell a story about family and chromosomes is to choose a beginning for a story that has no beginning, and an end where there is no end.

Theresa had grown up the oldest of five, in a Catholic family—first in Irwin, a small town outside Pittsburgh, and then, as her father ascended the ranks of the phone company, in the suburbs of Philadelphia. I had grown up outside New York. My father was deeply Jewish, and deeply nonobservant; my mother was technically Jewish, a wedding convert, but had grown up in Japan, arriving in America at the age of thirty.

Raised in the cradle of devotion, Theresa had become a chemistry major. She already had the best qualities of the scientist she would become: pragmatic, thoughtful, *observant*, in the secular sense. She liked organic chemistry. She was interested, she said, in the fact that tiny quantities of neurotransmitters made it possible for you to remember your name, or what happened yesterday. Over twenty years ago, and who knows what I said in response? Probably I sipped my tea, nodded vigorously, and did my best to continue appearing sensitive, since that was clearly working.

Having been brought up, myself, by pragmatic relativists—wanderers, loners, skeptics—I was trying to write poetry, the religion of the irreligious, and had developed an enthusiastic taste for absolutes. But every difference between us was part of a continental attraction. In late-night conversations interrupted by alcoholic braying from the dorm balcony, I made sweeping statements on topics I knew nothing about, after which Theresa would calmly ask a question I had not thought of or point out a fact I had not known. I kept talking, to keep her from going away. I had found someone I should not let go of. This perception has endured, beneath my boring turmoil.

We dated through college. In graduate school, in the days before cell phones and e-mail, we racked up three years of eighty-dollar phone bills, saw each other on alternate weekends, memorized the highways between Ithaca and Philadelphia. I finished my master's in poetry writing, taught English for another year, then moved to Philadelphia. A year later, in 1990, we were married in her parents' suburban church, with over two hundred guests, most of them from Theresa's side. We had added, to the standard vows, a promise "to honor each other's spiritual growth." The words were vague enough to be permitted, but different enough to startle the parish priest, who had been drowsing in a chair on the dais. The reception was a spectacular success, although the caterer had a panic attack and locked herself behind her office door. I played guitar, badly, with the band. Theresa threw the bouquet and garter, and children fought over them. By then my mother and father, who had looked uneasy and outnumbered on the hard pews, had begun to enjoy themselves. The next day, in a synagogue I had visited only once, we were blessed by a rabbi before a sparse assembly of immediate family.

We rented an apartment in Philadelphia, so Theresa could finish her degree; I taught freshman composition at three different colleges. Two years later, after months of fading hope, Theresa's father died of non-Hodgkin's lymphoma. A year later, Theresa finished her degree, and we moved to North Carolina. Theresa had a postdoctoral fellowship at UNC–Chapel Hill, and I got a job teaching comp at Duke. It was 1993. We bought our first house, a foursquare on two acres with a failing well. We got Penny, an eccentric and submissive cinnamon-colored mutt, and began to think about having a child.

A year and a half later, Theresa discovered, on her first trip to the fertility clinic, that she was already pregnant. "We do good work here," said the nurse, smiling. Two weeks later, my father called to say he had a spot on his lung. I immediately began renovating the house. Ellie was born that October, a pure happiness ringed by sawdust, end-stage cancer, and ungraded papers. My father died four months later. Soon afterwards, I quit teaching to raise Ellie full-time at home and write poetry when I could.

In 1998, when Ellie was two and a half, Theresa was offered a tenure-track job in Oregon. After our years living on the margins of academia—mobile, rootless, hypereducated, underpaid—we might, at last, settle down. Another dream of permanence, beginning with another departure. We visited in February, and as Theresa negotiated the equipment budget in her startup package, I took Ellie to an elementary school playground. Twilight, cool out but not cold, everything wet, a sliver of sunlight weighed down by clouds. I wiped off the dripping slide with my jacket. The trees, across the playground, were shrouded in pale green. That evening I asked one of Theresa's future colleagues: wasn't it early for spring leaves? No, I was told, that was moss. From all the rain.

So we bought a house in Corvallis, Oregon, where the ocean was on the left, the jays looked wrong, and it hardly ever snowed. We arrived in September and began settling in. We went to the Farmers' Market. We found the bagel place, the coffee place. In the evenings we went to Chip Ross Park, where you could climb a small rise and look south down the valley, a flat swath of grass and interstate. You could see glints of the Willamette River, in its wide meander north towards the Columbia. To the east were new mountains, abraded cones edging snowy tops above green foothills; beyond them were all the rivers I wanted to learn. To the west were the older hills of the Coast Range, rounded and blurred together like the waves of the Pacific beyond.

We liked the town; it seemed tidy without being sterile, free of the Southern social codes that had puzzled us in North Carolina. In Oregon, everyone seemed to be from somewhere else too, so we fit right in. We made friends easily. Theresa began teaching, setting up her lab, writing grants; tenure was not a given, but her chances, given reasonable progress, seemed good. We enrolled Ellie, then three, in a preschool. While she was there, I wrote and worked on the house. It was not long before we began, cautiously, to think of a second child. Ellie had been so wonderful, such a gift beyond imagining, that it seemed unfair to deny her a sibling.

Until Laura was born—or, more precisely, until her diagnosis—we could still understand ourselves as having a typical American story. We had grown up in the suburbs and gone to college. We had graduate theses bound in black, stamped in gold, and printed on archival paper, to endure for nonexistent readers. We had experienced the death of parents, the birth of a child. We did not attend church, or synagogue. We leaned to the left politically, but beyond voting did little. Now that story seemed over, and we seemed part of another one, where you spent your life in hospitals, you had to sue your local township so your kid could play soccer, and you got airlifted in the Lifeflight helicopter, once in a while, to a major medical center. We did not feel ready. We had, as one friend e-mailed us, taken an exit ramp to another planet.

We had not only lost our own story, but the possibility of *any* story. A story, in its very structure, offers comfort. Even the bleakest story has a curve of action—a beginning, middle, and end—and so it offers the possibility that experience can have an intelligible shape. But having a child with Down syndrome did not map onto a rising or falling curve of action; the event derided every curve. It spoke of chance, not continuity—in the original meiotic error, by which the extra chromosome came to occupy an egg or sperm, and now, in the array of dire probabilities the pamphlets disclosed. So we felt clueless, benighted, deceived. For months it had been true. We had not even known what our story was.

We sent away for books: *Medical and Surgical Care for Children with Down Syndrome*, *Babies with Down Syndrome* (in *The Special Needs Collection*), *Differences in Common*. I lifted them like prophecies from the Styrofoam peanuts. At night, long after Ellie and Laura had fallen asleep, Theresa and I lay side by side, the space on the quilt between us scattered with papers, reading. I had the new-parent guides and pamphlets, Theresa had full-text article printouts from her Medline searches: *Down syndrome* AND *heart surgery*, *Down syndrome* AND *anesthesia*. She read quietly, intently. I interrupted her, every five minutes or so, with a statistic, an anecdote, a random thought.

Starved for knowledge, I gorged on information. I read about dental hygiene, leukemia, mitral valve regurgitation, special-needs trusts, mainstreaming and inclusion, physical therapy, communication skills, atlantoaxial instability. I felt like the students I'd taught years before. A term paper was due, and I had just discovered how much there was to look up.

Laura slept quietly in the Portacrib beside our bed. We draped the pink horsey blanket over the crib, to keep the reading light out of her eyes.

My desperate cramming had its roots in a simple fact: *I had no way to think about Down syndrome.* I did not have a thesis, concerning Laura. Every approach seemed threadbare. I had been wondering, in my vague, science-ignorant way, about Nature versus Nurture. But Nature/Nurture seemed not a choice, but an opposition strained to the breaking point. On the one hand, the effects of Nature were obvious: the chromosome, the heart defect, delayed development. And yet Nurture would make the difference, according to what we were reading, between a child who might graduate high school, and a child who could not tie her shoelaces.

There is little I would change about the books I was reading. They were reasonable, occasionally wise. And reading them, I became fluent in a wisdom I did not possess. I had read, for example, that Laura was "a child first." I repeated it to Theresa. I tried it out. It sounded wrong when I said it—though, more exactly, it sounded wrong and right at once, not quite accurate but also deeply true. What did that mean, *a child first*? If she was *a child first*, then what was she second? The idea seemed not to go far enough. I didn't want *a child first*. I wanted a *child*. I wanted some sliver of Laura's life left pure, not claimed by medicine and experts. I wanted an unencumbered happiness. Not happiness with footnotes, caveats, and codicils, not the attenuated, saccharine, me-too version of the real thing, but the thing itself. We had experienced it with Ellie, instinctively, easily; with Laura, we would have to learn it. Or she would have to teach us.

I gnawed at consolation. In a parable of acceptance known universally among parents of children with Down syndrome, Emily Perl Kingsley writes that having a child with Down syndrome is like booking a trip to Italy and landing in Holland instead. "It's just a *different* place," she writes. "It's slower-paced than Italy, less flashy than Italy. But after you've been there for a while and you catch your breath, you look around. . . . And you begin to notice that Holland has windmills . . . and Holland has tulips. Holland even has Rembrandts."

But it is not like arriving in Holland, at all. It is like waking up to the same world you went to sleep in, except that overnight a team of industrious demons has jigsawed your picture of the world into a ten-thousand-piece puzzle. You know that you will be piecing things together for a long time, and that when you are done the seams will be evident everywhere.

I read "Welcome to Holland" to Theresa.

"Welcome to Holland," she said acidly. "More like welcome to Croatia."

Every piece of advice, no matter how reasonable or well intended, seemed remote, like distant shouting. I ticked off every noun in every sympathetic pamphlet: anger, yes, grief, yes, disappointment, yes, check, check. Yet the feelings seemed attenuated, distant, not mine. This too was a part of the script: shock, numbness. Check. It was vaguely disappointing. My feelings weren't original, only diluted. As for the future, I assumed I would also feel grateful, loving, and well adjusted, eighteen years down the line—a naturalized citizen of Holland—but in the meantime, Theresa was red-eyed, my stoicism was fraying like a rope bridge, Ellie was desperate to help and desperate to please, and Laura's heart, according to the ultrasound, was basically a Swiss cheese of holes and malformed valves. But we coped. We tried not to let Laura get too upset. We tried to pay more attention to Ellie. We e-mailed updates to friends and family. We kept reading.

What I found myself turning to were the brief, anonymous accounts transcribed from parent interviews and reprinted in *Babies with Down Syndrome*. The transcripts had not, like "Welcome to Holland," been polished into wisdom; they seemed questions, not answers. They did not package experience into parables or lessons. They did not presume to say what I was feeling, or what I would feel, later on. They did not reassure. And I found they made me feel better. They were often stark: "I wanted people to say congratulations, and they didn't. It was like my baby had died." "When the doctors told us at the hospital that our son had Down syndrome, we both just thought the world opened up and swallowed us right then." And while they offered hope, they were also honest about the limits of transformation: "My daughter is going on two, and I still think about the fact that she has Down syndrome every day. I'll think, 'Oh, she really looks (or doesn't look) like she has Down syndrome right now.' Or, 'I wonder if she's doing that because she has Down syndrome?' Or, 'Wow—she seems so smart and inquisitive; how could she have Down syndrome?' I don't feel especially sad when I think these things, but I guess I haven't really accepted her Down syndrome either."

There is a thread of sentiment in many of the writings about Down syndrome, an indigestible, treacly sweetness—Marilyn Trainer is a no-nonsense, welcome exception—and in the beginning, in particular, I could not abide it. I still shy away from the roses, the angels, from the rhetoric of Holland.

But beneath that sentiment, often enough, is a toughness earned from years of facing down a skeptical or outright hostile public. Emily

Perl Kingsley, and others in her generation, and the generation before her, were the pioneers; if we have an equilibrium now, if we have come to accept our children in a matter of weeks rather than years, or at all, it is because of them, both for their political efforts in changing the landscape of disability, and for their personal efforts, their witness to the raising of their own children.

It is a remarkable experience to read memoirs from the mid-twentieth century. Remarkable, first, because of how *little* has changed. In Lucille Stout's *I Reclaimed My Child*, for example, the chapter titles with the exception of the first—could be stations of my own journey:

1. My Child Is Sent to an Institution

2. I Have an Opportunity to Learn about Mongolism

3. I Reconcile My Knowledge about Mongolism with My Feelings about Having a Mongoloid Child of My Own

4. The Mongoloid Child Can Fit into the Family Picture

What is different, though, is that the journey takes *years*, and that the child—institutionalized in early childhood, a secret that warps the family—never comes home. She lives at the institution; the happy ending is that she comes to meet her parents, to know them, and to visit them on holidays.

Stout's memoir is about finding words in a vacuum. It takes years to even find someone who knows something about "mongolism," to work up the courage to speak with him; it takes even longer to begin to articulate what she has been feeling, to share her feelings with her husband, and to lurch towards an acknowledgment of her child. The loneliness of the experience is unimaginable. There are hardly any words to find, no memoirs, no Internet, nothing, and so the journey is larval and slow. She describes the enormous difficulty of acknowledging her institutionalized child. Of training herself to say that she has three children, and not two.

Parents like Stout are the discoverers of Holland. We have a different difficulty: we arrive in a country where everything is already built, where there is little left to discover, and where preprinted slogans are ready to recite. *A child first.* We struggle to find words against a muffling acceptance. Because the right words already exist for us, our spoken messages, in the beginning, tend to outstrip the unspoken. We arrive before we arrive.

No matter how sane, accurate, and up-to-date my sources were, there was one way in which research was basically futile. The knowledge I needed was rooted in experience, not literature. One reason it was so frustrating to read Emily Perl Kingsley was that she was writing from the other side of acceptance. I was just not there yet, and no story or statistic could get me there.

You can no more know what Down syndrome is like from research than you can call yourself a sailor after looking at a depth chart. To see a neatly inked *47* is very different from being at sea.

We had found out, from a blood test, that Laura did not have leukemia—chances were one in a hundred, which seemed, after the improbable fact of Laura herself, almost likely—and the heart, I was warily confident, would be fixed. But late one night, I read that the life expectancy for a child with Down syndrome was about thirty-five.

I set the book down and looked around the room. Thirty-five, that'd make me seventy when she died.

"You can't go by those numbers," said Theresa. "That probably includes infants who died early."

I nodded, but said nothing, slackening inside, resigned. Endless work, just to get her to functional adulthood. Then early Alzheimer's would set in, and then we would mourn her.

I was thinking a lot about the late stages of Theresa's first pregnancy, and the early days after Ellie was born, when my father was dying of lung cancer. He'd been pronounced terminal when Theresa was two months pregnant. As Theresa swelled towards her third trimester, my father, with each monthly visit north to New Jersey, diminished, his thin frame approaching the skeletal. Every feeling seemed fused with an inexorable mitosis, the sure duplications fueling both happiness and grief; the tumor seemed a parody of our growing and unborn child. Now, five years later, we had another beginning haloed by trouble.

It was wrong, I knew, but I could not shake the feeling of familiarity. Just as I had after my father's diagnosis, I was spending time on the Web, scything through prayers and digital roses, clicking and scrolling towards an inedible harvest of terms. Whether with Down syndrome or cancer, I saw that at the core of the medical condition was a negotiated, endlessly interpreted, but finally unchangeable fact: a metastatic cancer, an extra chromosome.

I talked my way through it, as I always do. Theresa listened, as she always does. But when I began saying how similar things were, this time around, what with the new baby, the medical, the microscopic, the uncertain future, Theresa interrupted to say that things were different now. "Cancer was bad news," she said. "Down syndrome is only hard."

Faultline

Laura was three weeks old now, closely monitored, fragile but stable. She had a mild case of jaundice—a failure of the liver to break down bilirubin—which, given her other problems, seemed like a vacation, an ailment you'd take on just for laughs.

Bilirubin breaks down in sunlight. But it was mid-March, still too cold to spend time in the weak winter sun. So Dr. E. had given us a special vest lined with sun-temperature bulbs. It was black, heavy, military-looking, with a thick fiber-optic cable, like a tail. We'd slip it on her, click the cable to the light source, flip the switch, and an intense green light would emanate from her neck and sleeves.

She looked like a baby Borg, from *Star Trek: The Next Generation*—a guilty, geeky pleasure of our childless twenties. The Borg were pale, remorseless, humanoid drones. They sailed around the galaxy in giant cubes, making everyone join their personality-free Collective. "Resistance is futile," they intoned. "You will be assimilated."

She lay glowing in the Portacrib.

"Resistance is futile," said Theresa.

"You will be assimilated," I said.

People were, for the most part, incredibly kind. They were concerned. They offered help. They struggled to say something appropriate. That struggle, and not unkindness, characterized most of our interactions, and it seemed appropriate that a disorder so specifically affecting language should bring people to the edge of words. You could see it in people's eyes: they had no idea what to say. And yet *something* had to be said, if only to avoid the silence.

Some glossed her difference in religious terms—she was an angel sent to teach the world love; she had been assigned to us, meant for us, somehow. Some filled in the newborn blank of personality with qualities like "sweetness" and "happiness." Some looked to the future, to a life that could be, with help, "full" or "productive." I smiled tightly and said little. Every consolation invoked its opposite: the idea that she had been destined for us, or intended for us by a greater power, papered over a demonstrable genetic randomness; the mantra that "they" were "sweet" seemed a desperate grasp for "normal" features; the "productive life" seemed a consolation prize for someone all but barred from a *reproductive* life.

We heard both that it was good they didn't know they have Down syndrome and that it was sad that they were just smart enough to know. We heard that Laura would always, in a way, be a child, and we heard about adults living in their own apartments. We heard about second cousins, deceased aunts, grade school classmates, children of neighbors: a faint constellation of distant stars, their light arriving from long ago.

She was elusive as a particle, a quark in the cloud chamber of rumor. She was flash, trace, implication. She could not be observed directly. I collected the world's responses to Laura, I plotted them on the vague graph paper of worry, and in the end no curve appeared. There was no pattern to what people said, so I could arrive at no general theory of Down syndrome in the world. Some people were okay with Laura, some were obviously thrown, some were intensely uncomfortable. Beyond the fact that she exposed the assumptions of everyone who met her, I could not say much.

It was not the words, anyway, that seemed most significant. It was everything around the words that seemed most telling, the mute expressions, the body language, the eyes, and it was these I learned to trust. Though I could not assent to Dr. E.'s belief that Laura had been meant for us, neither could I miss the decency and kindness that informed his words.

In the end, I rejected every interpretation because I needed to find my own. And yet everything I said sounded as wrong as everything I heard. Writing poetry seemed equally pointless, and like a sailor watching the ship leave port without him, I simply let it go. It was strange, how easily it had slipped away. For years, I'd jury-rigged a life to make room for poetry. But I could no longer stand the idea of fussing over line breaks, of spending days on a stanza. Like everyone, I was at a loss for words.

We walked everywhere, pushing the new stroller our friends had pitched in and bought for us. We tucked the blanket around Laura, let her sleep in the sun. We'd stop at the park, so Ellie could swing on the monkey bars. She'd taught herself how the summer before, practicing until her hands bled. Now she was learning to skip a bar on her way across.

One day, she got invited to the birthday party of a friend she hadn't seen in a while. Pure chance: both parents stand talking, eyeing the Impromptu Playdate Dynamic, and after a while one says, "So, we're having a little get-together this Saturday . . . " As often happens, Theresa took the girls, so I could have some time to myself. When they arrived, Theresa felt underdressed. There were moms in full makeup and pearls. "At parties like those," she said later, "I always feel like the one oddball chicken who gets pecked to death."

As it happened, she was only ignored. So she was present more or less invisibly when a pregnant woman shared her test results: "We just got the results of the amnio back," she said, "and the baby is *normal!* I was so relieved that he wasn't going to have six toes or anything."

It was a Down syndrome moment. To have a child, any child, is to thrust ordinary mysteries into the foreground: mortality, love, inheritance. Any child excavates the latent. But to have a child with Down syndrome is to push those pleasant mysteries into more difficult territory. In moments like these, the question is always whether to speak up. Whether to acquiesce. Theresa said nothing. It was a party for someone else's little girl. There was no need to ruin it. When she came home and recounted the story, I said, "You should have introduced her to Laura."

I said some other things too. I ranted until the anger ran out, and then I only felt defeated. It was pointless to rage against a joke that in the Pre-Laura Epoch, only a few weeks before, I might have made myself. We had found ourselves on the other side of a faultline: our child was different, so our lives were different too.

Each time I shared the news, I faced the difficulties of narrative. There was no way to tell Laura's story. There were only two incompatible scripts. The first began with a chromosome, flowered into abnormality, and ended with a family's ruin. The second narrated a child with challenges that were overcome in the end. One seemed brutal, the other sentimental, and neither really seemed to apply.

So I had begun to cobble my own script together. In it I tried to be frank about the difficulties we faced, but to insist on hope. I talked about Laura attending kindergarten one day, in the regular class. I said how Ellie was doing. I never said the word *angel*, and if I made jokes, they were loopy, edgy, or both. And because the existing scripts starred either a generic child or a human mistake, I tried to say what was only true for us. When I talked about Laura's heart defect, for instance, I'd say that I'd once worked as a medical transcriber for a pediatric cardiac surgeon. I'd seen him operate, and I'd learned that fixing hearts *was* routine, something that happened every day.

I always included the detail that did not appear in any parent narrative or pamphlet or guidebook I had seen: the confusion over Laura's eyes. I explained what little I knew about the history behind that confusion. That the syndrome is named for John Langdon Down, the

Victorian physician who discovered the condition. That Down had noticed the distinct appearance of one group of patients at the asylum he
ran, particularly about the eyes, and decided that those patients, all
ethnically white, had somehow "degenerated" in the womb. They had
assumed the features of another race. Since the contemporary term
for "intellectual disability" was "idiocy," Down called the condition
"Mongolian idiocy." His patients were "idiots of the Mongolian type."

Down's label was twisted, weird, and deeply wrong. And yet, for
precisely those reasons, that label was oddly reassuring: even though
"Mongolian idiocy" named both my ethnic identity and my daughter's
diagnosis in a bizarre and horrible way, its difference from the clinical-
sounding "Down syndrome" suggested that progress had been made.
As far as I was concerned, Down was a crank, a racist, a historical footnote. If I thought anything else, I would not have mentioned it to anyone. The point was not that Mongolian idiocy had anything to do with
me; the point was that it *didn't*. So the label, paradoxically, became a
term of reassurance.

At the same time, that label was far from a distant memory. Everyone
had heard it. One friend, telling her parents, had discovered that they
did not know the term *Down syndrome*, but on hearing *Mongolism*
lit up with recognition. So the term, and all its variants—*Mongoloid*,
Mongolian—became part of the script, which worked well for most
interactions. But it failed when I called my mom, when it collided with
an older script between us.

We hadn't told her about the diagnosis yet, though we'd called her
from the hospital once Laura was named. She'd been pleased, though
she had said, reproachfully, that Laura's name was hard for her to say
(one *l*, one *r*), and besides, it was the name of the First Lady. While I
knew the news of Down syndrome would make these matters trivial, I
wasn't looking forward to her reaction, and I knew I was already pissed
off enough at the world not to handle it well. So I kept finding reasons
not to call.

Still, friends knew. Acquaintances knew. I had to call her.

She was, like most people, shocked by the diagnosis, doubly shocked by the heart defect. As per the script, I reassured her. "Kids with Down syndrome go to school these days," I said. "In regular classes." I also told her about the heart defect, which was hard to spin in any remotely positive way, but I quickly offered reassurance. "Remember that surgeon I used to temp for?" I said. "Ross Ungerleider, the guy in North Carolina? He did these surgeries all the time, like two a day. This is routine, these days. It'll get fixed. It's going to be hard but it'll be fine."

My mom was doing okay up to this point. For her. She was on the edge of panic; I could tell she would be up late, chewing the news over. And that is the point where I should have ended the conversation. I should probably not have gone on to tell her about the confusion in the hospital over Laura's eyes, and the condition's historical name.

"What?" she said.

She was born in 1927, and her adolescence had featured starvation, sewing uniforms for soldiers, and the firebombing of Tokyo. Twelve years after the war ended, she came to the United States to study English, stayed to marry my father, raised me and my sisters in the suburbs of New York, endured years of slights from cashiers, mechanics, realtors. Her entire life was involved with the racial divide implicit in the term "mongolism"; it was, literally, the ocean she had crossed. So she then understood, I think better than I did, the implications of the word.

I pushed on with the script, trying to reassure. To clarify that so far as I then knew—Laura was a month old—"mongolism" belonged to the bad old days. That prejudice was gone now.

It was too late. "'Mongolism,'" she said. "Why would you *say* that?"

It dawned on me, too late, that she had taken offense. It was not an outcome I had imagined, *could have* imagined, before I called her. That she would panic, that I would need to reassure her, I expected. That the word would spark a reaction, I should have anticipated. But that she could see me as aiming the word *at* her was literally unthinkable.

That my mother is Japanese, that the world and the war she came from is a part of me—a part of me, in every cell, a part of the air as I grew up, a fact beneath and before the names—has always been a source of pride. When I was a boy, I'd decided to start calling my mother *O ka san*. The word had defined a slim but real connection to my origins, a pride in what I was, a reminder. It was like saying *itedaki-masu* before we ate, or *gochisosama* when we were done eating, or saying *Itemarimasu*, "I'll be back later," when we left the house.

So while I didn't imagine us sharing a good chuckle over that wacky Victorian doctor—John Langdon Down, him and his racial theories!— I also did not imagine the way things would go. What "mongolism" misnamed was what we shared.

Later that day, my mother called back. "*George*," she said, with the hushed urgency I long ago came to dread. When my mom says my name in that way, she is about to say something she cannot help saying. I cut off the conversation quickly. An hour later, another phone call. "*George*." She had spent the last hour doing research on the Internet.

"The extra chromosome always comes from the mother," she said.

I knew this was not true. The likelihood of Down syndrome increases with maternal age, but sometimes the extra chromosome is carried by the sperm, not the egg. I also knew why my mom had seized on this fact. If the chromosome came from the mother, it didn't come from her side of the family. She could not be blamed.

"It doesn't," I said.

"It does," she said. "I read it somewhere. It always comes from the mother."

"That's not true," I said, my voice rising. "It comes from the father sometimes, and anyway what does it—"

"Yes," she said. As if I had not spoken. "I read it. It's true."

"*It doesn't matter where it comes from*," I said. "She's here *now*. We're not blaming anyone. It's no one's *fault*."

I wished my father were alive, to say *No, Ranko, that's not how it works. It's just genetics.* But the idea would continue to preoccupy her. Later that year, in another phone conversation, she would return to questions of inheritance and cause. Ticking off her family history, she mused aloud about her half brothers, my uncles: "Makoto was starving during the war, but he turned out okay. Kazu is okay. Taka was okay." I had lost hope, by then, of explaining that chromosomal nondisjunctions are random events, but it seemed to me, even then, that Laura was okay too. Whatever her difficulties, I wanted my mother to accept her as she was.

But all that was still to come. In the moment both of us were silent.

It was then my mother announced that children with Down syndrome used to be given away for adoption.

After that, the shouting began. "Why are you telling me this?" I said. "What does this have to do with *anything?*" She was shocked. "*Of course* I didn't mean that you should have given Laura up, *no, no, no!*" I had misunderstood. The point was that things were better now.

It was not the first time we had argued. She had not approved of my choices, though they mirrored hers—to become a writer, and to take care of children at home—and the results, given a mother and son who are stubborn, and stubbornly alike, were predictable. That this history was now translated into the language of science, into chromosomes and "mongolism," only seemed typical of our new life. We were writing a new script, but we seemed unable to discard the language of error.

We had to explain Down syndrome to Ellie, so we sat her down in the darkened living room. She understood that something was up. We rarely make a point of a formal family meeting, and besides, Theresa had been in tears a lot lately.

I said, "Your sister has something called Down syndrome. It's not like being sick, but it does mean that some things will be different."

I felt flushed, saying this, as if I had been caught in a lie. Ellie was frowning and studying the carpet.

I said, "She might take a little longer to learn to read. She also might take longer to learn how to walk, and she might go to school a little later. Also, she's probably going to have to have surgery, because her heart has some holes in it."

"What's surgery?" said Ellie.

"It's when the doctors have to cut open your chest and fix things."

"Like when Penny had surgery?"

Penny, our dog, had eaten a pebble, and it had gotten stuck in her salivary gland. Her appearance after surgery—the white plastic cone, the shaved jaw, the long, stapled-shut incision—had made an impression on Ellie.

"Right, exactly," I said. "Except I don't think they'll use the big ugly staples on the outside."

"Oh," said Ellie.

"The main thing," I said, "is that she's part of our family and we love her."

"Okay," said Ellie.

And that was it. What for me was a statement made on faith, the right thing to say, something I knew to be true but would struggle to understand, began, for Ellie, as a simple fact: It's Laura, her sister. She's one of us.

At the end of April, the shock of Laura's diagnosis was wearing off, and we had begun to find a few certainties in the wreckage. What had once seemed an overwhelming responsibility was beginning to seem manageable. There had been the earthquake of the original diagnosis, and the single aftershock of the heart defect, but there had been no other news.

We were getting help from Benton County Early Intervention, the office that helps at-risk and "special-needs" children. We had an early intervention coordinator, a physical therapist, an occupational therapist. The coordinator, Pat Hill, had been an early ray of light; when

I called her to explain who we were, and that Laura had Down syndrome, she said, "Congratulations on the birth of your new baby!" The therapists were dedicated and friendly, and for them the diagnosis was nothing new.

It was all enormously reassuring. When Laura was first diagnosed, I had no idea what an occupational therapist was, let alone where to find one; now Gloria Wong, professional, friendly, affectionate towards Laura, was there to explain the pincer grasp, and Kate Layne, the physical therapist, could talk about trunk strength and balance. With them, and with Pat, we could begin to map out realistic goals. With their help, our burdens lightened a little: yes, there would be work, but the work could make a difference. Our efforts could help her.

In this light, even the heart defect was less daunting. It was operable. What had seemed an absolute sentence of nature now seemed susceptible to the efforts of nurture: not curable, for there is no cure for having an extra chromosome in each cell, but, in a way, treatable. Ameliorable. And then Laura caught a cold.

Early evening, and the downstairs shower was running, the door ajar. I didn't register it at first, and then noticed the steam. I went in. Theresa was sitting with Laura, watching her carefully. Laura's lips and fingernails were purplish, towards blue. She breathed with shallow gasps, her chest caving in.

The cold had come on quickly, the way it always does with children. Only the day before, she'd begun coughing, sniffling, emitting tiny cat sneezes. But this was different. We bundled the girls into the car, trying to hurry without rushing. We dropped Ellie off at a neighbor's and drove to the emergency room. A nurse taped the oximeter sensor to one toe and frowned at the reading. Then she got another sensor. A doctor came in and looked at the number. Then he set the oxygen at one liter and admitted her for observation.

What looked like a bad cold was actually a respiratory virus, complicated by Laura's heart defect. Because of its holes and incomplete valves, the heart was already overworked: blood leaked across the ventricles and atria; it murmured backwards up one-way valves, mixing oxygenated and deoxygenated blood together. To compensate, the heart pumped harder. Now Laura was congested, and since babies, at nine weeks, breathe mainly through the nose, her oxygen intake was down, which forced her heart to pump even harder.

We waited to be moved upstairs. Laura was doing a little better, with the transparent tusks of the oxygen cannula hooked into her nose. I sang "Oh! Susanna" to her, mixing up the verses. Its weirdness was soothing somehow, its shocks of humor and dream and dire circumstance, trouble and joy impacted in a rhyme:

a buckwheat cake was in her mouth
a tear was in her eye
the sun so hot I froze to death
Susanna, don't you cry

'She needed an X-ray. The technician and I took her down the hall to Radiology. In a dimly lit room was a Pigg-O-Stat, a special restraining device for infants. It had a sort of bicycle seat made of clear green plastic, and two curved plastic doors with leather straps. The seat was mounted on a circle of plywood, which rotated to provide the camera with front and side and back views. The plywood was cabinet-grade: I remember noticing the thin plies on the platform's edge, finished to a lacquered gloss.

We sat Laura down and strapped her in. I thought of the early days of photography, heads braced in iron clamps for the long exposure time. I did as I was told, raising Laura's arms straight up, like a dancer in a Broadway musical. The tech swung the doors shut and tightened the straps. Laura was screaming, which was good, since her lungs would be inflated for the exposure. I could see her skin flattened against the plastic, like something underwater. The tech hurried back and aimed the camera: a bright light with a cross of shadow appeared on Laura's chest. The tech centered the cross on Laura's heart, easing the camera into position on its heavy articulated arm. Then we tied on lead aprons and hurried out of range. Click, hum, and then adjustments for lateral and dorsal views. We got Laura unstrapped and I eased her out, consoling. We headed upstairs.

The X-ray film showed clouds, uncertainties against the hard arc of bone. There was fluid in Laura's lungs; she was in partial congestive heart failure. Only now did I learn that the phrase referred to congestion in the lungs, not the heart. Another day, another fact. Laura, by then, had been placed in a "mist tent," heavy plastic curtains draped around her bed, her body swathed in an Albuterol-laced fog.

After two days, the local hospital decided Laura would be better off somewhere else. Our town is not large enough to produce many children with Down syndrome. Of those, only one in four would have a heart defect of this severity. Of those, only some would get this sick, and of that smallest pool yet, many would go straight to Portland in the first place. Laura's situation required a pediatric cardiologist, which the local hospital did not have. Although Laura's care was good, it was also becoming obvious that she needed to be moved. Theresa had overheard the nurse on the phone with the attending, saying, "This little girl needs to be up at Doernbecher. She should not be here. You better call right now because I don't want her crashing on my shift." When the attending came in, he smiled and said, "We think she'll be fine, but we'd like to send her up to the children's hospital, just as a precaution."

"It always amazes me," said Noah, "how little there is to a house. Look at it, just three and a half inches of stud and some sheathing. Nothing at all between you and the outside, if you think about it."

It was the summer before Laura was born, and we had just torn out the big picture window from the smaller upstairs room. I'd been smart enough to hire a carpenter this time—Noah, a neighbor and friend, who chain-smoked hand-rolled cigarettes, drank espresso like water, and punctuated each sentence with short karate chops, one hand against the other. Noah later moved to Iowa City with his family, where he opened an espresso hut called Zip Drive.

I leaned out of the hole, looked down at the yard with its construction trash: scraps of tarpaper, pink insulation, sawdust, hunks of old framing sawed out clean, nails and all. It was like being in a treehouse. You could step right out the window and go down the extension ladder. I climbed down to cut two-by-fours. Noah called down measurements; I came halfway up the ladder to hand him the pieces, and he nailed them in. The nail gun made a decisive, vowelless sound, like punctuation without words. Every now and then the compressor kicked on in the shed, satisfyingly loud.

This time, I had promised Theresa, things were going to be different. This was partly a matter of atonement, not only for previous projects, but for the house itself, which I had chosen. By the time Theresa had been offered the Oregon State job, she'd burned through her vacation time and sick days, doing interviews. So I'd flown out to Oregon, toured our new town with a realtor, and seen seventeen houses in a day. Theresa and I had done our best to coordinate the effort over the phone, but in the end I emphasized two viable choices, the soulless ranch house with the nice yard and the bungalow with "character"—a realtor's word that glossed over the sheer ugliness of the low-beamed addition in back, the cat smell, the indeterminately ochre carpet, the fist- and foot-sized holes puncturing the drywall, and the small, sloppily painted mural in an upstairs bedroom, where an angry sun and moon smoked enormous joints in a cloudy sky. It was a project, I admitted this. But the house had a wired shop.

Now, two years later, I would get to the upstairs. I would repair the drywall. I would paint over the mural. In the bathroom, there would be tile, matching fixtures—the toilet, bathtub, and sink were three shades of Seventies goldenrod—and a skylight. I would convert the upstairs rooms into bedrooms: we'd have expanded closets, trim, new windows, and pine built-in cabinets in the eave walls. Banks of drawers for clothes, open shelves for books and games. We could free up the downstairs, I told Theresa. We could double the effective size of the house. Besides, I reasoned, once the new baby was here, we would be even more strapped for time than we already were.

But all my reasons were decorations of an impulse. I wanted a saw-blade blurring into maple, dust flecking my wrists and lungs, the slop of joint compound, the give of solder sweated into a copper tee. I wanted these things without knowing why, as if I had woken up with an itch to sacrifice a goat.

It was all depressingly, exhilaratingly familiar. Six summers before—when we still lived in North Carolina, when Theresa was pregnant with Ellie, and my father was dying of cancer—I had decided to renovate our kitchen; and after planning each detail on graph paper, I'd taken a wrecking bar to the walls. There were the wires and pipes, the old heart pine hidden behind lath and plaster: the house's anatomy, real, subcutaneous, assailable, a system I could change.

Theresa's brother, Mike, came down for the summer to help. He'd had a busy year of being sixteen years old, and it was thought a spell of hard work with his brother-in-law might be healthy for him. But the weeks with Mike were probably more useful to me. He was good company, levelheaded, averse to complication. His and Theresa's father had also died of cancer, two years before. We didn't talk much about it, but the situation was reversed now: Mike was clear-eyed, the older one. Absences swirled around us, as real as sawdust. We set up the radial arm saw in the living room.

In July, we turned off the water so we could plumb the kitchen sink, and after three days of this, Theresa's tolerant, mock exasperation began to fray. It was ninety-five degrees outside. She was six months pregnant. She had survived the nausea of the first trimester, the sawdust and solvents of renovation, my incessant thinking aloud about various construction options, not to mention the vertiginous mood swings of an about-to-be father about to lose his own father, and now she was showering at the gym and doing dishes in the bathtub. She was scrubbing plates like a pioneer, with cold water carried in a bucket from the well, and she said, "Okay, *enough.*"

She had had to make several other things clear to Mike and me, like the need for regular hours. We tended to start work by driving to Bullock's Barbeque for lunch, where we downed large plates of vinegary chopped pork, baskets of hush puppies, and endless refills of sweet tea. By the time we rolled out of Bullock's into the scorching afternoon, dropped by The Home Depot to exchange the wrong size plumbing fittings we'd bought the day before, and driven back to the home/worksite, it might be three o'clock. So when midnight came, we were just reaching our peak levels of productivity. Theresa would emerge in her nightgown, smiling, and say brightly: "Okay, boys! Enough with the drill!" "Okay, okay," we'd say. It was a good dynamic: we were irresponsible, and Theresa corrected us. So she would go to sleep, and we'd go get a video before the store closed, keeping the volume low, snorting over movies like *Fletch* and *Billy Madison.*

Once a month, I drove north to New Jersey, to the warren of chocolate-colored townhouses where my parents lived. With each visit, my father was a little thinner. We had awkward conversations of the kind we were supposed to have; we read the *New York Times* over bagels and lox; we walked to banked mailboxes through a sickly, New Jersey-sized ration of woods, following an asphalt path about fifty yards along a creek. It emerged at a parking lot by the community building, pool, and a tiny pond whose grassy borders were smeared with goose shit.

I'd take my father to the hospital. He'd stand on the scale, and the oncologist would slide the heavy chrome weight into the 150 notch: too high. He slid it back to 100, and then slid the smaller weight across, until the needle of the scale wavered, an impossibly slow vibrato. My father was six feet tall, 132 pounds. The oncologist said: "Paul, you're wasting away." He had the bedside manner of the Angel of Death. He was from India, and my mother distrusted him. "We should get a new doctor," she'd say. "We should get a second opinion." My father would shake his head and say, "Ranko, it won't make any difference."

During the summer visits, my father's death still seemed far away. Though there was no hope of cure, it was still possible to sit and trade sections of the *Times* over coffee. It wasn't a deathbed vigil: that would come later. For now, my father didn't look that different. He moved a little slower; he still had his wits about him; some of his hair had fallen out, but as we made sure to point out, he was bald anyway. There were flashes of what was coming, as if an X-ray were strobing on behind him. He would vomit, suddenly, uncontrollably. Once he doubled over in pain, thinking he had broken a rib. Cancer made the bones brittle: we'd been warned this might happen. He stayed bent over in his chair. "Jesus," he said. I urged him to go to the hospital, and my mother said, "Paul. *Paul.* Listen to George." He shook his head; after a while, he said he was feeling better. "It's all right," he said.

Before the end of each long weekend, I was ready to leave. It was never easy; in a sonnet I wrote later, I compared the feeling to the acceleration of a plane leaving the ground, the propulsion forward, the undertow of gravity. I knew that, back in North Carolina, surrounded by the ruins of renovation, I would feel the gravitational pull of my parents' house, and that as long as my father lived I would be caught between two homes. And yet I was beginning to understand what my marriage had announced, and what this event would etch a little deeper: that the phrase *my home* had come to refer to a little thousand-square-foot box in the North Carolina piedmont, and *my family* meant Theresa, and whoever would arrive in late October.

That fall, Mike went back home for his senior year of high school, and I returned to my job teaching freshman comp. The kitchen was functional, not finished: the cabinets done but doorless, raw edges of drywall and WonderBoard everywhere. On weekends I chipped away at the blank spots. Theresa was tired more often, and when she stood on chairs to reach for reagents on high shelves, the Scottish postdoc in her lab scolded her, told her to wait and got them down.

On a sunny September afternoon, my father called to say that he was about to die. He thought he had about five minutes left, and he wanted to say how much he loved me. His voice was slurred, as if he'd just been to the dentist. I sat in a house in the middle of North Carolina. I was almost thirty-one. I had papers to grade. About an hour later he called back. "Sorry, George," he said. "False alarm."

When Theresa came back from work, she held me for a long time, and that was a comfort just deeper than loss.

On one of my last visits north, I drove my dad to the hospital, took him to Radiology, where the X-rays that were meant to slow the cancer, but also made him nauseous and weak, were aimed at his hip. He walked slowly into a shielded room. Over the door a red light came on, then went off. When he came out, he said, "You know, I don't know if they're really doing anything in there."

Good Samaritan had called Doernbecher Children's Hospital, ninety miles north in Portland. Doernbecher would send down the PANDA team, an ambulance with respiratory specialists. They'd be here in a few hours. Theresa would ride up with Laura, and Ellie and I would follow later that evening. There was nothing to do but wait.

So I took Ellie home and decided to tile the tub surround. We packed overnight bags, put them in the car, took the cordless phone upstairs, and mixed up a five-gallon bucket of mortar. Ellie handed me tiles and spacers. I cradled the phone on my shoulder and made arrangements for the dog, setting tiles as I talked, row after orderly row like a calendar of stone. As Ellie and I left to follow the ambulance, driving north on I-5 and counting hawks on poles, the half-completed job was already curing in place, turning to rock above the unplumbed tub and scattered tools. And for months, the bathroom stayed exactly the way I'd left it, like a diorama in a natural history museum: these are the tools they favored. This is the way they used to live.

Border

We arrived in the evening, winding uphill towards the hospital, an ey-rie of glass overlooking Portland from the southwest. On the way up you could see glimpses of the city through the trees. I pointed out the lights to Ellie.

Strange now, to remember how good it felt, how much like an ad-venture. We had a new family member who'd been transported to the hospital in the big city, and I was glad to be the dad, reassuring Ellie that Laura would be okay. It was like being a kid again, when you won-dered when anything exciting would ever happen, a terrible accident or emergency to make everyone feel sympathetic, admiring, glad they weren't you.

We found a slot in Patient Parking, left the Subaru ticking over the stenciled Raggedy Ann-like face of the hospital's logo, slung duffel bags over shoulders, walked towards the entrance with its fountain. The glass doors slid open onto a soaring atrium that smelled of coffee. We found our way to the elevators, went up to the ninth floor, found the room number Theresa had given me.

Laura was in a raised bed, asleep. Her breathing was labored. There was a narrow bed by the window, a brown vinyl-covered reclining chair. We made our way around to the window, where Theresa was sit-ting. We set down our bags and tried to stay out of the way.

Her last IV site had failed. It had been a struggle at Good Samaritan to get her IV sites started and to keep them viable. She was univer-sally acknowledged to be "a tough stick," and by the time she got to

Doernbecher she'd already been through the ankle and wrist sites. But she needed fluids. One nurse began inspecting the pale webwork of veins at Laura's ankles, her wrists, her scalp. She said she felt like a chimp at the zoo, grooming.

Ellie saw this was going to be dull. She began drawing.

One resident wanted to give Laura epinephrine to help with her breathing.

"Won't that speed up her heart rate?" I asked.

The resident looked blank. Suddenly I realized she was younger than we were.

Ellie said she was tired. We unfolded the recliner and pulled a sheet over her. Instantly she fell asleep.

They gave Laura the epinephrine and began work on the IV. And like any sick nine-week-old being held down and repeatedly punctured, Laura screamed. The nurses were sweet, apologizing, saying they knew how hard it was on the parents, and we said, it's okay. It was okay: she needed fluids. But they could not find a good vein because the IV sites were used up, and because, since Laura was beginning to get dehydrated, her veins were even smaller than usual.

Laura screamed and screamed. They held her in place and said soothing things. They parted the sparse hair of her scalp. They slipped in a needle, looking for the thin dark line of blood, a solid line striping the sterile tube, but every hoped-for gusher was a dry well, or a drop or two, tapering to nothing. Laura's cries had overtones of every tiny animal I'd ever heard, fallen nestling, mouse in trap, shrilling guinea pig, and the nurses were sorry but they had another site to try. We were past smiling, but we said, Go ahead.

It went on for ninety minutes. I had no precedent for this. I felt stretched thinner than phyllo dough. I remembered the time when we'd let Ellie "cry it out," listening to her howl from the next room. That sound unstuck time: I remember wanting to go to her and comfort her, and sticking it out, and checking my watch after five minutes, convinced it had been twenty. This was like that, except not. Theresa had bright spots of color, high on her cheekbones. She had the expression of someone who is choosing not to burn holes in the wall with her eyes. Like me she was doing what seemed rational, which was to choose to trust the people in the room.

Nothing worked. They did their best; they couldn't find a new site. In the end they left, and turned up Laura's oxygen setting to three liters, a steady hiss that whispered *sick, sick, sick* from the wall. Laura lay in the bed, propped on pillows, lips parted, chest heaving. Her heart rate was 180. I had never seen her so completely exhausted, distressed, pushed past the edge of some endurance I could not imagine.

I didn't know if we'd done the right thing, if we should have set a time limit, if we should have spoken up and said, That's enough. I didn't know whether it was a good idea to give a child with a damaged heart epinephrine and then overload her with stress and pain. I still don't, not being a doctor, but I do know that, had I to do it over again, I would've stopped the process far sooner. I would have said, Enough. I would've asked for the name of the best IV therapist in the hospital, the one who gets Saturday night off, and asked to schedule an appointment with that person. I would've asked how much difference it made, whether the IV went in then, or the next day, or at all, and would've asked to balance those events against the cost of pushing Laura to the point of needing three liters of oxygen. But we were then learning how to advocate for Laura, and advocacy requires calm and tact, and we were still recovering from the first shock of Down syndrome and the second shock of the heart defect and the third shock of Laura's hospitalization, and we were strung out and sleep deprived to boot.

In the quick-anecdote version of that evening, we emphasize the fact that Ellie—the littlest insomniac, the girl who didn't sleep through the night till age five—slept like a rock through the entire ordeal.

— ◆ —

When we woke up the next morning, Ellie wanted to go back home. So Theresa and I began our new routine. One of us would sleep in the recliner by the bed, the other on the window seat. In the morning, I would leave at six and drive the ninety miles back home to Corvallis, where Ellie was staying with friends. I'd spend some time with her, take her to preschool, check messages, get fresh clothes, drive back in the afternoon.

Back in the hospital, I washed my hands raw. I took the elevator to the Starbucks concession in the lobby and stood in line with red-eyed parents, nurses on break, doctors craning at the readouts on their beepers. I drank black coffee, at any hour. We were awake half the night anyway, listening for alarms or interruptions in breathing; and the room was awake too, lit by the dimmed lamp over the bed, the orange numbers of the oximeter, the fluorescence that seeped in under the door. There was never total darkness, and never a total, enclosing sleep. In the daytime, the lights stayed on, buzzing faintly, a tinnitus of the unresolved.

We were helping Laura heal, so she could get to heart surgery in one piece. That was the story, as we understood it. But inside every story, another story is beginning.

I got the phone call at home, in a blur between walking the dog and dropping Ellie at a friend's house. It was Theresa; a nutritionist had come to the room, bearing a chart and a recommendation.

"She said Laura was failing to thrive," said Theresa.

"She said what?"

"Actually," said Theresa, "she said, 'Did you know that your baby was failing to thrive?'"

The nutritionist had been delicate, but pointed. No trace of warmth. Her disapproval was almost tangible.

"Of course she's failing to thrive," I said. "She's in the goddamn hospital."

Failure to thrive, as I later learned, has a definition: a baby falls across two bars on a standard growth curve. The nutritionist had brought a curve to show Theresa where Laura was, and where she was supposed to be. But Theresa, as a working scientist, deals with curves all the time, and though she was shocked, she was skeptical too. The nutritionist had the wrong growth chart, one used for typically developing children. Children with Down syndrome grow more slowly and tend to be shorter; they have a different growth chart.

"Did you tell her she used the wrong chart?" I asked.

"It didn't matter," said Theresa. "She wants us to put in an NG tube."

"A what?"

Feeding problems are chronic; the need for food is immediate. The infant who forgets how to eat and needs months or years of therapy to prod her memory awake, still needs nourishment in the meantime. For this reason, clinicians depend on the NG tube. "NG" stands for "nasogastric." The nasal end of the tube, the foot or so that hangs out of one nostril and is taped to the cheek, has a port that flips open to admit medicine and fluids. The other end is pierced to let fluids drip out; it threads into the nose, down the esophagus, and into the stomach.

Though Laura had lost weight, she hadn't stopped nursing. So Theresa refused the tube, hoping that as Laura's health improved, her appetite would increase, and her weight would follow. With that decision, our experience of the hospital began to change.

We've seen our share of hospital dramas—*ER* was a bad habit for a while, at least until flaming helicopters started falling on unpopular characters, and every character slept with every other—and so we knew the TV version of conflict. But that's not how things were, in actual life. On TV, everything would be magnified for dramatic effect. In Theresa's place would be an inappropriately calm, peasant-skirted mother with nontraditional opinions about vaccines and a devotion to breastfeeding at the expense of her child; in mine, a businessman in denial, rushing to work while his child languishes; and in the doctor's place, a rugged yet sensitive male model, trying to make the family see reason. For us, things were less dramatic, more complicated. Theresa wanted to breastfeed, but she wasn't ideological about it; she was the voice of reason, not hysteria. I felt an occasional protective anger for Laura and Theresa, but I didn't yell, and I didn't storm into offices. As for the clinicians—the resident, and then the cardiologist, also wanted us to put in the NG—none were models, and none fell into the tidy boxes reserved for TV characters.

So our interactions never rose to the level of drama. They couldn't, because with few exceptions, we liked the people we dealt with, most of whom were competent and friendly. Besides, the characters kept changing. The nurses were on eight-hour shifts, and they rotated from patient to patient. After the weekend, the doctors changed as well. We felt like ceremonial monarchs: powerless, subject to a slow parade of visitors, each approaching our room at every hour of the day or night, each with a different request, a different opinion, a different message about what "the team" was doing. We heard a great deal about the team, but never saw them all at once. We did figure out, before long, that the cardiologist outranked them all, so we learned to appeal to him, but he wasn't always available. We also learned the hard lesson, as Laura's chart thickened past the point of a quick read, that although we were the most medically ignorant of Laura's caregivers, we were the only ones who knew the whole story. We got good at giving each newcomer the condensed summary: list of medications, newfound allergies, condition of recent diaper, amount of oxygen, most recent decision about the tube. Our life felt less like *ER* than a medicalized version of *Groundhog Day*. We were trapped in an unfinished story.

The disagreement over the NG tube was marked not by conflict, but by a maddening lack of specificity. Theresa wanted to know what happened if things went wrong; she wanted a plan to help Laura learn to eat again. Instead of a plan, she got reassurance. She was told the NG tube was not particularly invasive, that parents loved it because it made things easier, that it would only be in for a few days, that it would not be uncomfortable for Laura at all. True, perhaps, for other parents, but not for us. As it turned out, Theresa's intuition was correct: NG tubes can have profound effects on an infant's feeding patterns.

What was frustrating, much later, was to find that this was widely known. Doing research for this book, I came across a *New York Times* article profiling the psychologist Ramasamy Manikam, who runs the New York–based Center for Pediatric Feeding Disorders: "Underlying [Dr. Manikam's] work is the notion that eating is a learned behavior, not an instinctive one. Babies fed by tube after birth may never learn to associate the sensation of hunger with the act of eating; babies who do not move to solid food by the age of 8 months may not learn to breathe, chew and swallow without choking. When those learning opportunities are missed, children can develop a deep anxiety that defies logic, something that Dr. Manikam compares to a fear of flying. He has spent a career trying to break down that fear, most often in children with disabilities who become accustomed to tube-feeding early in life."

I don't know, for sure, what Laura's doctors were thinking. But I think we had a conflict between the long-term view and the short. The doctors were thinking in the short term. They were looking at a child with a respiratory illness and a serious heart defect; their goal was to get her well and keep her well until surgery. As far as we could tell, they considered issues of feeding to be secondary. Get the calories in her, get her well enough to go home, get her through surgery in a month, and dish off the long-term problems to early intervention and the primary care physician. Heart first, stomach second. We saw this logic, but for us, the short term was a prelude to the long. When the surgery was done, we wanted Laura, as far as possible, to be able to eat normally. Her burden of acceptance would be lighter if she could break bread with others. And eating—nursing, then moving on to solid food—would be crucial preparation for speech, which would also be more difficult for her. Eating was a crucial component of Laura's future in society, a future that was vague, unpredictable, and much on our minds.

Over the next few days, the question became not whether, but when. Laura had nursed indifferently, holding steady—not declining, not improving dramatically—but when she showed the first signs of dehydration, we reached a compromise. We would attempt to feed Laura for one more night. If her weight gain continued to be sluggish or nonexistent, we would put in the NG tube the next morning. At four in the morning, we woke to the riffling of a chart and saw the silhouette of shoes beneath the door crack. A nurse came in with a plastic packet, saying she had orders to put the nose tube in. It was almost perverse: there had been nighttime visits, but they had been quiet, discreet. Angry, blurred by sleep, we sent the nurse out of the room's dark into the perpetual light of the hallway. In the morning the attending pediatrician came in and said, "So. I hear you refused the NG tube." And despite her tone of accusation, we had to accede: Laura needed to gain weight. She stayed in the hospital for five more days. After we got home, she was healthier, heavier, her stomach filling reliably with pumped-in breast milk; but even as she gained weight, her appetite was tapering fast. One night, about a week after we'd gotten home, Theresa heard a faint clicking in the back of Laura's throat as she nursed. The next day Laura stopped eating by mouth.

After a few days, Ellie had wanted to be with us: the novelty of consecutive sleepovers had worn off. I was glad to have her back. We roamed the hospital complex together, buying a keychain in the gift shop, ice cream in the cafeteria. Ellie lit up with gratitude, as is usually the case when Strict Dad is evicted by Fun Dad, and I was dazzled, as always, at my luck. We stayed up late watching TV. Ellie snuggled with Theresa, while Laura slept. One night, Ellie and I left the unit, walked down the corridors in our socks, and stood on the glassed-in skybridge, looking east towards the lights of Portland. On the far shore of the Willamette, I could see the glowing sign of the Museum of Science and Industry.

I began to notice the other children. I noticed Ellie noticing; she seemed observant and unsure. In the hallways were two boys racing wheelchairs. One was bald, his arm bruised from needle sticks. A Child Life Therapist wrung her hands and walked quickly after them, saying, "Boys, boys, please slow down." Out in the enclosed courtyard, I saw parents with smiles like weathered wood, walking behind two- and three-year-olds who laughed as they toddled after beach balls, the clear plastic tubes trailing behind them to IV trees. The infusion bags had names like cisplatin, vancomycin, Taxol. Pacing the halls as Laura slept, I saw rooms decorated for the long term: 'N Sync posters, crepe ribbons, Christmas lights.

We'd been learning, for eleven weeks, what our life was; the children's hospital accelerated our education. In coping with the grave minutiae of our daughter's illness, we were absorbing the deeper fact of change. We had ceased to resist the situation. Although we often felt damaged, stressed, fearful, we no longer felt completely lost: Laura was our daughter. We would manage. And being in the hospital had helped us realize we weren't alone. There, at least, we were no different. We felt—not at home, exactly, but a sense of belonging, of common cause. We'd met Stacy and Johnson there, whose son, Elijah, was born two weeks after Laura, and had the identical diagnosis: Down syndrome, AV canal defect. We could compare notes on cardiologists, or talk about feeding tubes, just like parents in the park on Saturday, talking about new teeth and first steps. It was nice, not having to explain.

We were beginning to see her, our second daughter. The single soft loop of hair that stood up most of the time, only lying flat when she was really sick. Her rare smiles—they were still events, something you'd mention. The occasional wide, happy O of the lips, as if she wanted to speak, but was unsure what to say. Her eyes, newborn blue, towards sea green. Her quick, inexhaustible, furious temper, flaring with every failed IV stick. I saw it whenever we tried to put the nose tube in.

Back at home, she took two naps a day. I stood at the bedroom door, listening for her breathing. Sometimes, hearing a soft rustling, I'd go in to find her already awake, inspecting the ceiling. I'd jar the mobile for the last wound notes of Brahms's lullaby, the soft colored dinosaurs rotating a quarter turn; I'd clown above her, making faces, and as she saw me, she'd open her mouth wide, track my expressions, reacting, taking it all in, alert, *thinking*. Animated, radiant in shadow, with the blinds drawn against the afternoon.

This Is Eating

May 2001

I assemble my materials: surgical tape, stethoscope, antibacterial lubricant, NG tube with wire stylet, child needing supplemental nutrition.

I set Laura on the changing table. I tear open the plastic packet and remove the nose tube. I grease the end of the tube with antibacterial lubricant, then tear off a few lengths of tape and stick them to the rail of the table. Then I brace a forearm lightly across Laura's chest and arms, pinning her in place, and start pushing the tube into her right nostril.

I keep threading. Laura flicks her head from side to side, making choked sniffling noises, her face red, eyes squinched shut. I am waiting for the blue dot marked on the tube to reach her nostril. It helps to thread the tube in quickly, but it's important to pay attention. I have in the back of my mind the embarrassment of a friend's pediatrician, who deftly pushed the tube in, saying, O.K., eighteen, twenty, twenty-two, Got it! All the while the tube was steadily uncoiling from the child's mouth.

I withdraw the wire stylet, then tape the now-limp tube against one cheek. I get the tape as close to the nostril as possible, and I don't leave any slack. Laura will probably pull the tube out anyway before the week is up, but I don't want to make it easy for her.

I get out a ten-milliliter syringe and the cheap yellow stethoscope the hospital sent home with us. It looks like a party favor, but it works. I place the stethoscope's disk above Laura's stomach, below the heart, my right side, her left. I draw about five milliliters of air into the syringe, open one of the ports on the tube, insert the syringe's end into the port, and blow. I hear the faint *pfft*, which means I've placed the tube correctly. I think of the nurse in the hospital, who told us not to worry, that if we placed the tube in the lung the child would turn immediately dusky. She had only seen it happen once.

It was a difficult time. The oxygen concentrator, which dribbled an extra half liter of oxygen into Laura's nasal cannula at all hours, thrummed like a diesel and smelled faintly of cigarette smoke, a residue of the last emphysema or lung cancer victim to rent it from the medical supply corporation. Our house smelled like a hotel room, and our lives were newly fragile: in the old days, Child with Stuffy Nose had meant, at worst, an ear infection and a course of amoxicillin. Now we tiptoed in fear of an avalanche. Laura's surgery would happen in a month, if all went well, if she gained weight, if she didn't get sick. If. Behind the days, an endless murmur of worry.

In the longer term, I was beginning to glimpse a future beyond the medical. In the first few weeks, we could still choose not to disclose Laura's diagnosis. We told people anyway—partly to hear ourselves say it, and partly because we knew we needed to claim the fact. But some days we didn't feel up to it. We just wanted to go out with our cute baby, heart defect or not, and keep things to ourselves. Now that option was closed: with the NG in, and a portable oxygen tank rattling around behind us, all the oohing and ahhing vanished, and the worried glances and gawking took over. Laura was a marked child. Everywhere I went, I could feel the pattern of stares forming around me, like iron filings around a magnet.

On some days I almost didn't mind. I'd feed her in the Starbucks, which entailed mating the nose tube to a veterinary-size syringe, filling the syringe with breast milk, and jamming the plunger in top to start the drip. I'd eye the sinking meniscus, watching Laura for signs of gagging; if she got too full, she would throw up. Then I'd refill the syringe.

It was performance art: everyone around her with their three-dollar coffee drinks and pastries, sipping and chewing, experiencing the rush of sugar, caffeine, of *consuming*, and here was a cute baby with a white liquid draining slowly into one nostril. I felt like putting up a sign: THIS IS EATING. People would glance up from their tables and pause a second longer than they might have, or slow down as they walked past the plate glass window outside, like cars passing a highway wreck, and though the entire change in my life, my family's life, was condensed into that stutter-step and pause, I didn't look up. I fed my daughter. I was a sensitive, competent stay-at-home dad enjoying a morning out with my special-needs child. I would pack up and leave when I was done like any other customer. Once, though, Laura yanked the tube from the syringe, dumping a precious ounce of breast milk in her lap. I rushed to stop the spurting milk with my thumb, knocking over my grande coffee and nearly scalding my daughter.

I was beginning to learn what Laura meant in the world. Though I may have begun to accept that difference for myself, I was still learning what it meant to others; and shame, protective worry, and a selfish concern for my own future difficulties blended together in an ongoing reverie, an inner argument whose terms never seemed fully defined. In this disorientation I turned towards the practical. Whatever "normal" might mean or come to mean, and wherever Laura might fall in the estimations of others, I wanted her to belong, to attend public schools in regular classrooms, to play soccer, to go to birthday parties. We would give her the extra help she needed; we would teach people to see her as a child.

The nose tube shadowed that vision. When others saw Laura, they registered her as different, and despite myself, I saw her as different too. The tube seemed almost parasitical, a worm of separation; with its swath of adhesive tape, its flotation-vest yellow, it literally defaced her. It made a sideshow of us wherever we went, and filled our days with conversations I increasingly saw as intrusive and did not want to have. In the medical realm, it was purely a means to caloric intake. In the social realm it was something else altogether.

Several months later, when our desperation had deepened without result, a neighbor came up to Theresa and said seriously, "You know, breast-feeding is really the best thing for them." She advised Theresa to "offer the breast," as if this was an option we had not considered. I wasn't there, though I can imagine the precise smile that accompanied Theresa's response.

She and Laura had been evicted from Eden. For nine weeks Laura had eaten instinctively, thoughtlessly, nursing until her lips slackened around the nipple; Theresa would detach her gently, as she had with Ellie, and lower her into the crib. It had been the last link to a normal childhood, and now it was gone. Sometimes, as Laura slept in her car seat, her lips suckled faintly against the air.

We had acquired a breast pump. It had two plastic discs, like futuristic weapons. Theresa pumped late at night and early in the morning; in the refrigerator was a row of dated bottles. When it was time for Laura to eat, there was another pump, a squat electronic box on a silver tree, and a case of plastic bags for the milk. We'd string up the bag on a silver branch, empty the warmed milk into the bag, wind its long tube through the pump's black wheel, connect the nose tube, and set the milliliters per hour; its creaky whir would begin, the black wheel kneading the milk in, drop by drop. We fed Laura on the schedule recommended by the nutritionist, bolus feeds during the day and drip feeds at night, the slow intermittent turning of the pump diluting our sleep and making our dreams vivid, restless. Sometimes the milk would clot or the tube would kink and the machine would start beeping, like a garbage truck in reverse. We'd start from dreams of botched surgeries and childhood houses to the red letters flashing FLO ERR, and we'd grope for the START/HOLD button to halt the noise for ninety seconds. I'd shake the covers loose, unkink the tube, and restart the pump. Sometimes it took three tries, the beep returning just as we drifted off; finally one of us would get up, get a new bag, warm up more milk, start over. Awake, seething, I thought of every child I knew, lulled at the breast, turning from it sleepy, content, drunk on love.

For Theresa, it was ten times worse. It was visceral, personal. She was the one whose body had been supplanted by machines. She was the one who had heard and felt the click in Laura's throat, and known. She and Laura had been intimately linked in the act of feeding, and it was her body that had changed in response to Laura's signals, each hour and each day. In comparison, I was a nutritionist.

We began to disagree. We replicated, within our family, the divide in the hospital. I was thinking about Laura's heart; Theresa was thinking about eating. She developed an unshakable hatred for the nose tube. She worried aloud that Laura would take years to learn to eat, that she had simply lost her suck reflex. I kept saying, It's only temporary. Wait until the heart operation. Everyone says there's a dramatic change. She'll get the nose tube out then. One thing at a time.

But after a while my consolations began to sour: they became rote, then impatient, then angry, then absent. I was tired of hearing about it. A bad heart could kill her; inability to eat by mouth would not. And I was used to Theresa's being the stable one; I was the moody one, yawing out of orbit and then settling back. I could be rocklike, steadfast, but only for short periods of time. Other trials—my father's lung cancer, her father's lymphoma—had united us, in grief and endurance. But this was different.

I studied the heart. I explored the Latinate-mathematical wilderness of gated ion channels and fluid dynamics and QRS complexes and Purkinje fibers. I read as if reading could change things. There was, however, no optimal depth of knowledge. If I saw the heart as a simple matter—as plumbing, a pump—then the plumbing could leak, the pump fail. If I delved into the details, then each one made the heart seem more fragile. I could be lost at sea, or lost in a labyrinth. It didn't really matter.

As Laura's surgery neared, we tended to the minutiae of waiting, submerging ourselves in a life now normal, now utterly surreal. We bought a plane ticket for Ellie; Grandma, Theresa's mom, would take care of her, first here, then for a week in Pennsylvania. We filled out unpaid leave forms, set up an Internet account in Portland. We ate takeout Chinese off paper plates; Laura ate with us, the infusion pump whirring breast milk into one nostril. We exclaimed over Ellie's newest drawing; we forbade her to touch her sister. We listened to Laura's breathing; we watched the color of her lips.

We broke down and got cable. We said it was for Grandma, but it was really for us. We were tired of poor reception for everything but PBS, and felt strongly that we needed the gentle, healing glow of mainstream stupidity to get us through this rough patch. It was one of the perks of our situation, along with not returning calls or e-mails if we didn't want to, ignoring the wrecked upstairs bathroom, and—for me, the crowning glory—canceling the extraction of my wisdom teeth. Having a child with a heart defect has little to recommend it, but it is an excellent all-purpose excuse. Ellie, who regularly went days or weeks at a time without TV, was agog before the hyperkinetic wonders of Nickelodeon and the Disney Channel. Theresa, watching *ER*, was glad to see the expressions of the doctors, free of static at last.

As the family Puritan, in spirit if not in heritage, I would set stern limits during the day, then grant myself slack-jawed hours at night. Slumped in blue light with a biology textbook, surfing the five hundred–plus channels of the Digital Silver Package far into the wee hours, I illuminated the cardiac cycle with Top Ten Lists, sports bloopers, *Seinfeld* episodes, and the interminable scrolling of the TV Guide channel, its numbered boxes advancing like the edge of an enormous gear. I'd hit the MUTE button and let the listings cycle through, as I read about less evolved creatures with no need for a four-chambered heart. The sea sponge, for example, which simply rooted itself in nutrient-rich waters, and absorbed whatever the currents brought it.

By midnight, the commercials got noticeably shabbier, as slick, effects-laden microdramas for cars and soft drinks yielded to amateurish spots for mattresses, recreational vehicles, debt consolidation loans, and 1-900 party lines. Around two, the infomercials would begin slithering into view, flashing their white teeth and rock-hard abs, and at last I'd turn the TV off. Padding into the darkened bedroom, I'd step over the oxygen and feeding tubes. I tried not to wake Theresa or Laura, shutting the door behind me.

I hadn't talked much with my mom, though I'd told her about explaining Down syndrome to Ellie ("*What? You told her?* Oh no, George. No.") But now she was coming to visit. She'd been in Japan while Laura was in the hospital. She'd meant to head back to New York, but at the last minute, she'd added a stopover on her way back to meet her new granddaughter. She would be with us for three days.

Her plane was due from San Francisco in the late afternoon. I clicked Laura's car seat into the Subaru, buckled Ellie in, and drove down Route 99W towards Eugene. In May, the grass fields are bright green after a winter's rain; there are fields of mint, a little darker, and in between the long straightaways, the road arcs slowly, like an asphalt shadow of the Willamette. The only car stereo we had then was a boom box, but I clicked in a tape, turned it on, and headed south. I drummed on the steering wheel, sang along, called out *TURN* as we sped through the big curve outside Monroe.

We parked and walked into the tiny airport and waited at the foot of the escalator. We could see my mom descending. She didn't look good—jet lag, I figured—but when she got to us she began coughing. Her eyes were bleary.

"This is a bad cold," she complained. "I must have got it on the plane. Other people were coughing too."

On an ordinary visit, I would have driven her home, asked after her visit, settled her in. I would have had Ellie show her latest drawings and play her beginning piano pieces. Then I would have taken her to Shogun Bowl, the Japanese noodle shop she likes. But this wasn't an ordinary visit.

"You have to keep away from Laura," I said. "She's having heart surgery in a month. She can't get sick."

She looked shocked. She looked like she felt the way I did.

We collected her suitcase. We walked out the sliding doors and past the taxis to the parking lot. We loaded her suitcase in the car and drove out. She tried to pay for parking, but I said no. I could see her, in peripheral vision, thinking it over: an occasional slight tilt of the head, a nod, her face set. We made small talk about her visit with her step-brothers, my uncles.

The visit went that way. There were no explosions, only tension. My mom was uncharacteristically abashed, almost contrite; I was clipped, cold, abrupt. On her last night with us, she asked if we could eat Chinese food. We went to King Tin, where the waitress kept reaching for Laura, saying *so cute*. We were polite at first, and then we just said no. You can't touch her. After an endless dinner the check came. My mother tried to pay and I said no. As we cleared the remains of dinner into polystyrene clamshell boxes, my mother stood apart, hugging herself a little, unsure what to do.

The next morning I drove her to Eugene in silence. I took her to the Horizon desk and waited until she was checked in. At the departure gate, we said restrained good-byes.

"Thank you for coming," I said.

She shook her head. She looked resigned.

"I shouldn't have come," she said.

One of the first things I noticed—after strangers staring at the oxygen tank, the collapse of the future, and the feeling that middle age had arrived early—was the absence of the apostrophe: in the United States, it is Down syndrome, not Down's syndrome. I had read, somewhere on the Web, that since John Langdon Down neither had nor owned the condition, the possessive was inappropriate. Similarly, the phrase "Down's kids" was frowned upon, since children should be thought of as individuals first. Over the years, I've come to agree. Laura is Laura, not a Down's kid. But I don't make a big deal of it. In practice, I've heard medical professionals and parents say "Down's" and "Down's kid," because it's shorter and more convenient.

I liked the confusion. If I said "Down syndrome," my hearer would likely assume the apostrophe was there, and I would know it wasn't. I felt like a native speaker, versed in tones inaudible to outsiders, able to hear presence and absence at once. Present, the apostrophe was Laura as we had suddenly, shockingly come to reconceive of her: a Down's kid, her life entwined with a condition inseparable from her humanity. It was the extra chromosome, the squiggle, the black mark that made all the difference. Absent, it was disability and deficit and defect, the hole in the heart, delays in speech, everything we would struggle against. There and not there, like the fifteen suspended days after Laura's birth when we knew and did not know, our worries and hopes flowering like blood cells in culture. A charmed and lost time.

It was a paradox to raise a child by. Down syndrome would have to be present and absent for us, or we would need to practice a presence and absence of mind. We would need to study Laura's condition, absorbing what we could of what was known, then set our knowledge aside. It would have to become, in the best sense, second nature. In the fullest knowledge of the forty-seventh chromosome, we might return to the old ambiguities of raising a child. I felt as if we had crossed a border in the dark.

Echo

Every time I opened a textbook or logged on to the Internet, every time I read *right ventricle* or *systole* or *sinus rhythm*, I felt a private embarrassment: these were things I should have known. Long before we'd moved to Oregon, before Ellie, before Laura, and before I quit the fractured, interim life of part-time teaching and office work to raise kids at home and write, I had spent a summer working as a medical transcriber for a cardiac surgeon. Every word had a seven-year echo.

The surgeon's name was Ross Ungerleider. He specialized in congenital heart defects, some of them "ditzel stuff," in his words, no-brainers requiring fifteen minutes to repair, and some severe enough to require a stepped series of procedures, as the child grew. Most of his patients were less than six months old. At the end of each operating day, he'd dictate his notes into a handheld recorder; my job, among other things, was to type up the notes. I'd sit wearing headphones in the windowless outer office, clattering out a dialect that was not yet mine—*hypertrophy, stenotic, Betadine*—and feeling, at times, like a medium: the voice in my ear droning its dream language, my fingers moving almost automatically, and the infants' stories spelling themselves out, in glowing letters, behind my convex reflection. I could tell the defect's severity by the length of the note.

On my first day, I got stuck on the word *mediastinal*, as in *mediastinal incision*—the initial cut down the center of the chest, after which the sternum is sawed or cut in half to expose the heart. I tapped the Dictaphone pedal, rewinding then going forward, like a teenager learning to parallel park. The word was a blur to me, outside the vocabularies I knew. If Ross had been saying *April is the cruellest month* or *Da capo al fine* or *1.9% APR financing* or *Fifty-five units shipped COD Scranton per usual*, I would've understood, but *mediastinal* was an aural smudge. I slowed his voice down until he sounded old. I sped it up until he sounded like a singing chipmunk. No luck. So I presented him with the draft, left the word blank, and asked. Oh, he smiled. *Mediastinal.*

He had wavy gray hair and walked in a kind of turbocharged amble, reflecting high purpose and relaxation at once. He had the confidence of someone who had already divided the darkness from the light and gotten most of the landscape sorted out, and apart from one very important last task, it was mostly a matter of having his archangels record the Latin names. He rarely got angry, but then people rarely failed to live up to his standards. He introduced himself to me as "Ross" but I called him "Dr. Ungerleider." If I was curious about a procedure, or a word's meaning, he was glad to explain. I remember saying that heart surgery seemed like plumbing, and he liked that, his eyes lighting up. "That's right," he said. "It's just plumbing."

I soon settled into the routines of the office. I wrote down new words on yellow Post-Its—*tricuspid, interventricular*—and stuck the Post-Its to the computer. I typed my first and only death note. I turned in my time slips. Delivering files to Cardiology and Medical Records, I learned to navigate the hospital's disastrous maze of color-coded areas, numbered floors, and cardinal points ("go to Floor 2, Orange Zone, South"). The hospital seemed a botched understanding of the body itself, physiology exploded into departments. I found shortcuts and blind alleys, less-used elevators and exits that locked behind me. And typing the record of children's surgeries, I began to understand what I was transcribing, to extract the arc of each story from the impersonal form of the op note, to see that behind name, medical record number, and the sequence of clipped jargon beginning *Chest prepped in the usual manner* and ending *Sinus rhythms resumed*, an actual child was

being, in effect, suspended: her heart stopped and packed in frozen sa-
line, her blood oxygenated and circulated by machine, until her inborn
defect could be repaired.

One morning I came in, and the anesthesiologist's secretary, with
whom I shared the outer office, was dabbing at her eyes. When I asked,
she steadied her voice, and said that _____, across the hall in the
pediatric ICU, had died. I didn't recognize the name. In the gentleness
of her voice was the implication that I wouldn't have. I didn't have kids
yet, after all. I was out of the loop: I was still the temp, and a childless
temp to boot. The story was off limits to me, like most of the hospital.
Though I was twenty-nine, I felt like a child myself, a tyke, my nose
pressed to the glass of the adult world.

In the fall, the job ended, and I went back to teaching. A year later,
Ellie was born into the hopeful ruins of renovation; four months later,
my father died. Soon afterwards, I quit teaching to stay at home with
Ellie. I'd written a poem about working for Ross, but beyond that, I
hadn't thought much about him. Then, in February of 2001, Laura was
born, her heart defect was diagnosed, and suddenly we were the parents I'd seen in passing seven years before, the red-eyed ones carrying
sheaves of forms. I'd been on the periphery of that storm, and now I
was at its center. As I began constructing my rudimentary, beginner's
map of the heart—oh, the atrium is the upper chamber; oh, the *right*
side sends blood to the lungs—I realized I knew nothing, nothing at all.
I could study all the textbooks I wanted, but on the morning of Laura's
surgery, I would simply be handing my daughter over to a stranger and
hoping for the best.

In May, we returned to Doernbecher for exams, an ultrasound, and
a meeting with a doctor I'll call Anna. We asked her about pulmonary
artery pressures, infection prevention, ACE inhibitors, mortality rates,
average postoperative stays, and the possibility of withdrawing the
NG tube before surgery to encourage Laura to breastfeed. They were
long and detailed questions, and Anna was clearly tired. In discussing

Laura's weight gain, she mistakenly said "ounces" instead of "grams," implying that Laura should be gaining nearly a pound a day. When Theresa pointed this out, Anna furrowed her brow over new calculations. But in the end, we only got the general sense that more calories were good. Eating, like Down syndrome, seemed a black hole to swallow clear answers.

"Do either of you have a medical background?" Anna asked politely.

We explained about Theresa's PhD in pharmacology, my work as a medical transcriber.

"Well, good," she said. "Do you have any other questions?"

"Yes," I said. "Who is her surgeon going to be?"

A softball. She seemed relieved. "His name is Ross Ungerleider," she said. She pronounced the name slowly, as if speaking to first-year medical students: *Tricuspid. Coarctation. Ungerleider.*

It was the same guy, the surgeon I had temped for, seven years ago. He had moved to Oregon only two months before, to head up Doernbecher's pediatric cardiac surgery unit. He was in the building at that moment.

Anna smiled as she left the room. "I'll mention you to him," she said. "It'll be interesting to see if he remembers you."

We gathered up our notes, pushed the stroller into the deserted waiting area. Laura was already asleep, exhausted by a long day of exams. Theresa began reorganizing the diaper bag, syringes and formula on one side, diapers and wipes on the other. She coiled up the loose nose tube, tucked the coil in an infant bootie, and pinned the bootie to Laura's shirt. On another day, I might've looked away as Theresa hurried, both of us treading worn paths towards a tense and familiar silence, but I was too overcome with good fortune to be resentful. I felt exhilarated, calm, at ease in improbability. I looked out the window, to the familiar view of southeast Portland and the Willamette River. Only two weeks before, during Laura's hospitalization, the view had seemed unreal: a diorama, toy bridges and buildings, a shoebox version of the world we'd been divided from. Now it seemed a landscape of the possible. Back home, Ellie was cutting intricate patterns from construction paper, waiting for us to return. I felt that my life, too, had been folded over on itself, snipped at random, then unfolded to reveal a strange symmetry.

It seemed that way for a little while. We drove away from the hospital, we sank into the landscape, and what had seemed neat and diagrammatic from above, proved a miscellany of detail up close. I clung to my diagram. I wanted the coincidence to mean something. But even as we drove south on I-5, and I prattled to Theresa about the fractal geometry of our lives, and she said, "Okay, slow down," I could feel the glow fading. I resisted. I was sick of weird news, sick of having our lives ruled by chance, by events that admitted no transcendent understanding. The extra chromosome had simply happened. So had Down syndrome, the heart defect, the feeding troubles: they had only happened, they were events without meaning, a life to accept, not understand. I could not abide this, so I worried the coincidence like a scab.

Back in Corvallis, I tacked the news onto Laura's story. It was a useful detail, a remarkable footnote, an exit from awkward silence; but after the initial exclamation of surprise, the coincidence produced a silence of its own, because no interpretation ever stuck. Every angel or fractal slid from its polished surface. It exemplified neither chaos nor pattern, it connected to nothing larger than my own, personal past, and so it did not sustain or console. It had been as radiant as a koan solved, and it was only the punchline to a seven-year joke.

It was June twelfth, the day before Laura's repair, a day of tests for Laura and explanations for us. We left Ellie with Theresa's mom, who'd flown west to help us. We got up early and drove north, the route familiar already. We walked from Patient Parking to the hospital entrance. It had only been two weeks since the cardiology consult, but it felt like years.

We lived like insects then, packing lifetimes of metamorphosis into days and hours. In the restroom off the main lobby, a viscous pearl of antibacterial soap in my hand, I knew I was absorbing the place's odors back into my clothes and skin and hair.

We stood in front of the receptionist until she looked up. We recited Laura's birthdate, produced our insurance card. We began to navigate the hierarchy. We chatted with the lab techs, waiting for a urine sample to appear in the plastic bag; we held Laura still as the IV therapist pressed a brilliant fiber-optic lamp against each of her wrists, then her ankles, inspecting the glowing territory beneath the skin. She withdrew a hot pack from her sagging purple apron, massaged it to start the reaction, held it against Laura's left ankle, and got her sample. We could have kissed her. We met with the cardiac nurse, who gave us the basics: a four- to six-hour procedure, then three to seven days in the ICU. She emphasized that these were estimates only. We met with an anesthesiologist, who tested even our appetite for bluntness and fact by saying, "Well, it's general anesthesia. Pretty much anything can happen." He handed us the consent form.

In the time between appointments, we paged through a white binder entitled *Your Child's Heart Book*. It contained pamphlets, a form letter ("Dear Parent(s): Your child has been diagnosed with a congenital heart defect"), and a pair of illustrations.

Both were in black and white. The first, labeled *Normal Heart and Blood Flow*, was Xeroxed from a textbook. It showed the atria and ventricles in cutaway, the four valves, the great vessels that received and distributed the blood. Inside each vessel was a curved one-way sign printed with the blood's direction: *from body, to lungs, from lungs, to body*, the simple circuit compromised by Laura's defect. The second illustration was an imperfect copy of the first. Compared to the textbook version, the heart of ESTREICH, LAURA R looked provisional, a sketch, a work in progress. Where *Normal Heart* featured the slick graphics of optimal circulatory health—its muscles dimensional with shad-

ing, its neatly separate chambers labeled in situ with custom fonts—
Laura's heart was all white space and line, its structures altered by hand
or mouse: the valves' cusps were ineffectual slivers, the septum reduced
to a few islands of muscle. Nothing was labeled. At the bottom of the
page, the parts of Laura's *complex congenital defect* were enumerated in
a short list, from *atrial defect primum* to *patent ductus arteriosus.*

I found the image consoling. In its starkness, it reinforced my tendency to see the problem as dire, but soluble: there were holes, Ross
would fix them, and ESTREICH, LAURA R would possess *Normal Heart.*
There were no gray areas: uncertainties, worries, the fears I lived by
were simply not mentioned. I saw all that as my own business, anyway.
So I was less receptive to the next item in the binder, a twenty-nine page
booklet called *To Mend a Broken Heart.*

To the extent that the book was simply written, informative, and
exhorted parents to Never Be Afraid to Ask Questions, it was useful. To
the extent that its illustrations seemed the work of a third-rate mall car-
toonist, to the extent that their grotesque caricatures of parents from
all ethnic groups faced the hard skull of death with demented, cheerful
denial, it was asinine and condescending. On nearly every page were
drawings that made *The Family Circus* seem naturalistic. Here was a
dad with an enormous, scrotal chin, holding his baby above a group
of sniffling toddlers. Here was a couple in the surgical waiting room,
the mom with a scribbled list of questions, her tongue stuck out on one
side, the dad checking his watch, his face torqued to a rictus of comi-
cally jangled nerves. The faces were bulbous, distorted, like balloon
animals. But grotesque as these were, they were eclipsed in absurdity
by the book's star: the cartoon heart.

It was identifiably medical and human, not a Valentine; it was pulpy,
thick, and muscled, and it had a severed three-branched aorta growing
out of its head. It also had arms, legs, pop eyes, and a diaper. It was probably male. It fingered the jagged line of an ECG; it sucked its thumb.
It stood on a table, holding a magic marker. A supine doll lay on the

table, its chest bisected by a thick line. Seated at the table were a nurse, evidently explaining, and a child, evidently listening. The heart wore a surgical mask. Its eyes were wide, staring at the doll's *mediastinal incision.*

On another day I might've just laughed. But in those days nothing was neutral. I wanted to help Laura. I wanted to face realities, to know survival rates and life expectancies. I wanted to *see* my life, and maybe, one day, to describe what I saw, to construct a clarity useful to myself and others. So the partial truths were worst of all. I tore at them like cobwebs, the cartoon versions of reality. They adulterated complex life, diluted it with the purity of stereotype. The cartoon heart embodied this debasement, with its googly eyes and diaper grafted onto muscle; and in its removal from the body, I saw a parody of the next morning's procedure, when Laura's *actual* heart would be disconnected, in order to be repaired.

In the very back of the binder was a plastic page slotted for professional business cards. It was a nice touch: the specialists had been fattening our wallets for weeks. I began extracting them, laying them out like a game of Concentration—the surgeon, cardiologist, cardiac nurse, lactation consultant, nutritionist, physical therapist, occupational therapist, speech-language pathologist, early intervention coordinator, developmental pediatrician, family doctor. I began to alphabetize. The act was soothing and absurd. I'd ordered a replacement box of business cards for Ross, seven years ago.

I slid in the cards neatly but ran out of slots before I got to *Ungerleider,* so I started over again, putting him first.

I didn't know if we'd actually get to *see* Ross. In the weeks before surgery, it became, for me, a test of the past's value: would we rate a meeting, or would he send one of his minions? Nor did I know what I'd call him: it had been *Dr. Ungerleider,* years ago, but then I thought: I'm thirty-six, and my daughter's having heart surgery. These seem to be tokens of adulthood. I'll call him Ross.

We saw him in the early afternoon. I'd remembered that he operated first thing in the morning, returning after lunch with a fistful of easy-listening CDs. When he walked into the examination room, energetic, hearty, firm of handshake, I felt as if I were looking through a stereoscope: the particulars of his face and voice and walk came back, and I was seeing two images at once, the past and present superimposed but slightly misaligned. The moment had depth, but its edges were blurred.

He seemed a little older, but not much. There was small talk for about forty seconds—the coincidence, when he'd gotten to Oregon, how old his kids were. Then it was on to Laura. He sat on the edge of the exam table, craning forward a bit, to where we sat in chairs. Okay, he said. And it was not unlike the old days, when I would sit in his office and we'd go over the day's priorities. There was a punch list. There was a purpose, which in this case was to inform the parents and to obtain consent. What he had to say was statistics, mainly: risk of complications, death, risk of surgery needed at a later date, risk of neurological damage. "We've made a lot of progress on that one," he said, "since you worked for me. That was—what, 1994?"

When he said "we" he clearly meant a community of surgeons, cardiologists, and researchers; and when he said "1994," he meant that year as a relative Dark Ages of cardiac surgery. There were quantitative measures of improvement. Mortality rates improved, complication rates lessened. He didn't seem to think about time and change much, not in the abstract, mournful, ruminative, poetic ways I have always both favored and tried to exorcise. He'd been too busy saving people. And the coincidence, too, whatever it meant, was not of particular interest to him. He enjoyed it, but seemed to ascribe no significance to it. It went in the OUT-box: there was a heart to fix. The atrial defects would be patched with GORE-TEX, the ventricular defect with peri-cardium, tissue snipped from the protective sac surrounding the heart. The tricuspid and mitral valves would be restitched for a better seal. The patent ductus would be closed, no longer patent. "Yeah, we'll just throw a stitch in that and ligate that off when we're in there," he said. Ditzel stuff.

We signed the forms that said we knew Laura could be injured or might die and that we had been informed of this fact. We shook hands again and Ross went out.

"There goes a man," I said, "without any self-esteem problems at all."

We toured the PICU. We signed a few last forms. We confirmed the op-erating time and Laura's feeding instructions: only clears after midnight. There had been a disagreement between the nurse and the anesthe-siologist, and we stayed until it was sorted out. Through it all we smiled and held our ground. We were learning.

In my old job, I'd seen the parents in the ICU, sitting by their kids' beds. I'd met parents who needed Ross's signature on insurance forms. They had the same deeply preoccupied look. They smiled wearily and explained the situation, the procedure the insurance company had balked at, and they knew Dr. Ungerleider was very busy but could he sign this to help them get preapproval? Behind the social niceties of consideration and greeting, you could hear the heavy gears of worry. And I could tell that all they wanted was for the trivia to resolve itself, so they could concentrate on being with their child.

And then we were back out in the sunlight. We drove down the hill; we were due back at six the next morning. Laura was first on the sched-ule. We were staying ten minutes away, at our friends Matt and Judi's house, and they were precise in their love and consolation, aware of the situation's gravity yet not overwhelmed by it, affectionate yet careful. We cradled Laura like a jewel. I drank a beer. We called home: Ellie was eating pizza with Grandma. In a few days they would fly back east to

Pennsylvania, and Ellie would see all her cousins. She couldn't wait. We turned in early, did a last tube feed, and set the alarm, as if it were possible to oversleep. I'd thought I'd be awake all night—I'm a stress insomniac from way back—but I fell asleep right away, and an eyeblink later it was just before five. We shut off the alarm before it woke Laura. It was dark outside, and we were as quiet as we could be, leaving the house.

In the ICU

It was 6:30 A.M., the operation was scheduled for 7:00, and the secretary behind the desk had no idea who we were. Behind her was a nurse, a man in his twenties wearing blue scrubs, a weary look, and an overnight growth of stubble. "Don't worry," he said. "We'll get you in on time."

We sat down, and in a few minutes someone said Laura's name as a question. We left the carpeted waiting area, with its lamps and magazines, for a room half-lit by fluorescent lights, its edges divided into curtained exam areas. We sat down and waited until a nurse rattled the curtain back. Late twenties, close-cropped hair, muscular forearms: a startling number of male nurses resemble ex-Marines. He weighed Laura, had us sign a last form, asked us about allergies. He explained what we already knew, that we would be in the surgical waiting room during the operation, and that the surgical assistant would come in with updates.

"Don't be afraid to step out for a minute, if you need to," he said. "It can get pretty intense in there. There are some families dealing with some pretty dismal issues.

"You folks are lucky," he continued. "This is a happy day for you. You're here for a repair."

Theresa had tears in her eyes, but she nodded, smiling.

They took Laura around the corner to the OR. The anesthesiologist had said, "Oh, she's so little, we'll just carry her." Theresa later told me that was the hardest part; it just made Laura seem more fragile. What I remember most of all is the gravitational pull of a possibility no one wanted to talk about. It competed with the pull of the earth. It made our own bodies feel different, knowing that Laura's was about to be cut open. I knew she could die and tried to understand that fact. Then I tried to forget it. We walked down the hall to the waiting room.

Soft chairs and couches, blond wood coffee table, the standard look of furnishings not meant for homes. A carpet patterned to hide stains. There was a telephone on the coffee table, and a few magazines: a twenty-year-old *House Beautiful*, a *Newsweek* from last year. It was as if someone knew that the day didn't matter, the year didn't matter, that waiting for surgery to finish is a no-time carved out of time, a boulder in the river. I found a current copy of *People*.

It took an hour and a half to get the IVs in. The nurse in the morning, the one who'd told us this was a happy day, had said, "Oh, they'll work on her for a couple of hours before he even washes his hands." Later, the anesthesiologist shook her head and said, "She's a tough stick."

This was the part where the op notes said *Chest prepped in the usual manner.*

The surgical assistant came in. "She's on bypass now," he said. "She's doing great."

"About how long do you think she'll be on bypass?" we asked.

"About thirty to forty-five minutes," he said. "Maybe a little longer. Any other questions?"

"I don't think so."

"O.K. I have to get back. Page me if you need to."

I turned back to the tribulations of Jenna Bush.

After several weeks on the job, I'd asked Ross if I could watch him operate sometime, and he said, "Sure!" So one morning I found myself in the OR—the place open to me as a temporary office worker, but forbidden to me as a parent. Ross didn't look up. The patient was a girl. Her head and legs were draped in blue, and I could only see the sterile field in glimpses, as bodies in blue scrubs moved in front. It was easier to watch the video monitor.

I stayed on the edges, talking to one of the nurses, careful not to knock anything over. I was wearing a disposable paper suit, like a giant FedEx envelope; it rustled against my good shirt and tie. Ross, bent over the child's heart, was completely absorbed. I felt totally irrelevant, a lurker, a voyeur. I didn't know the child. For me, she was a medical history number and a name I'd soon forget.

The nurse pointed out machines: heart-lung, anesthesia pump. I watched the monitor, something silver flashing against the wet mess of the body. I heard the high-pitched *rzzzzz* of an air tool. A bone saw, the nurse explained. "Boys and tools," she said, shaking her head and smiling. I'd remembered that, talking to Ross about Laura's surgery. He'd explained that Laura's sternum, at this age, was more like cartilage. You could just cut it, you didn't have to saw through.

The nurse said Laura was settled in and we could come on back. We followed, past rooms darkened for sleep, children unconscious beneath digitized vitals, and extended families red-eyed, talking in small groups, or staring up at monitors. The ICU was laid out, roughly, as a large square, with a central nurses' station ringed by individual rooms. Each room was partitioned from the hallway by sliding glass doors. Laura was in Room 10.

She seemed tiny in the bed. The incision stretched from just below her throat to just above her belly; I have blocked out or forgotten exactly what it looked like, having accustomed myself to the pale straggly line of her scar. I remember that her eyes were half-parted, filled with a kind of grease to keep them moist. She'd been given a paralytic to keep her from pulling out her tubes, and could not blink.

Her lips were taped shut around a thin clear hose. I didn't connect it, at first, with the ventilator, the squat machine that inflated and deflated her lungs for her, its screen drawing and redrawing a graphic of each breath. There was a catheter, which drained through a clear tube to a Lucite box graduated in milliliter increments. Arterial and venous lines looked magnified and apart under clear tape; pacemaker wires sprouted from her chest. Once I looked down and saw blood around one of the wires—it was "weeping," the nurse said—and I felt shocked, as if I'd been solving a crossword puzzle, and the paper had bled.

Above the bed, on an articulated arm, was the flatscreen monitor. It displayed her vitals: heart rate, systolic and diastolic blood pressure, right atrial pressure, left atrial pressure, pulmonary artery pressure, temperature, O_2 saturations. Each number was a different color. The numbers changed, moment to moment. Each readout had a set threshold; if her oxygen saturations, or "sats," dropped below 92, or her heart rate went above 180, an alarm would go off, a soft department store chime, echoed distantly at the nurses' station. We heard the chimes often. Usually it was nothing, but if the chime continued, the conversations would end. We'd watch together, Theresa, the nurse, and I, and if nothing improved the doctor would come in. We were already used to it, the way a ventilator's ascending trill or a flashing red number could haul you up out of waiting. Sometimes I would leave the ICU for coffee and return to see a knot of specialists at the foot of Laura's bed. From the back I could see them watching the monitor. I would come in and ask what happened and Theresa would say, "Her blood pressure crashed again," or "Her sats dropped again." Laura would stabilize and the crowd would thin. This, too, I got used to.

Across the bed from the monitor were the infusion pumps: for glucose solution, heart drugs, pain medications, sedatives. Each pump clutched a syringe. Each syringe fed a clear tube that snaked across the bed through a system of color-coded ports. The ports connected to Laura. Each tube had a flag of sticky tape on it that said WEDNESDAY. As the days went on, and the tubes were changed out, they accumulated new flags, until there was a confusion of days beside Laura's bed, a scrambled calendar: FRIDAY, MONDAY, WEDNESDAY, THURSDAY. A week without a year.

When I remember it now, I remember it as a single time, our time in the ICU. I collapse it, I confuse sequence, I travel by association across the days. But time was crushingly linear. We were waiting for things that had not happened yet. Laura had not yet come off the vent. She had not yet urinated in significant quantities. Her heart rate had not come down. Her blood pressure kept crashing, inexplicably. All of this imprisoned us in the present, kept us from an impossibly distant future when our child would breathe on her own. Though we knew she would, at the time it seemed unlikely. Her breathing without machines seemed part of our other life, the one visible through the picture windows that lined the hospital hallways. Out there, down the hill, was Portland, its traffic slowing at rush hour. Everyone down there driving and breathing.

In our bleakest moments, this stasis, this frozen waiting, seemed to distill the experience of raising Laura: the milestones stretching in an endless series, dominoes too heavy to fall. When will she breathe? When will she eat by mouth? When will she hold her head up? When will she crawl? When will she speak, hear, understand us? Every *when* seemed shadowed by an unspoken *if*. We had moved to the laid-back Northwest, where being "in the moment" is prized as a good thing, as something children remember and we have forgotten. But we were in the moment, and we didn't want to be there.

That night, Theresa went to Matt and Judi's. There was only a single bed in the hospital room; Laura seemed stable; Theresa was exhausted. Theresa said, "Are you sure?" I said, "Yes, yes, I'm sure, go get some sleep." It was around nine.

Then the soft chime of the O_2 alarm. I went around to the foot of the bed to look at the blue number. The alarm threshold had been set at 92, and the number was 89. The nurses looked too.

I could hear the corresponding alarm out at the nurses' station, like an echo from a distant wall: first the soft chime in here, then out there, its sound different, reverberant. Like birds calling to one another.

Now the number was 82, and both nurses were starting to move, their faces set. I backed out of the room. I started to call for a doctor, but he was already there. Others were coming in. The number was in the 70s. Other alarms were going off. The bright numbers blinking, lavender and kelly green and red. The ventilator alarm was going off too, its cricket's chirp rising. At the edge of the room I could hear the alarms above Laura's bed and then behind me a second later, and I stayed there, in between the sound and its echo. The number was 65, a number that had always meant equipment failure before. At this point my back was against the far wall of the hallway and I was thinking of *ER*, the TV show, the ritual revivals and urgent motions, actors above actors. I was not in a trance, exactly. I was awake, I was aware. On the TV show, the parents are always screaming and being ushered out quickly by a nurse. I tried to stay out of the way.

They had bagged her already and weren't getting anything, and then they saw that the oxygen tube at the other end of the bag had fallen loose. It was a new kind of bag, they'd just switched over. Ian, the intensivist, was saying, "I don't care what kind of bag, I need one on her right now," not shouting. The nurse hurried to the back of the bed, to the shelves where they stored the old kind of bag. She had to tear the plastic wrapper off it and come back around to the front of the bed, the hands reaching towards her, and then Laura was bagged again and they were squeezing the bag in the rhythm of human breath. Then whatever it was that had clogged the ventilator tube—mucus, debris in the lungs, whatever—got blown loose. The blue number started going up. The alarms subsided.

Ian stood at the edge of the door with me for a minute and told me Laura was okay. I asked if she had been without oxygen long enough to sustain brain damage, and he said he didn't think so. He smiled. As if to say, I know this is an earthquake for you, but around here this is no big deal.

I called Theresa and explained what had happened and said, "Why don't you come on back down to the hospital tonight."

Working for Ross, I'd crossed the hall to the PICU at least once a day, because that was where the coffee machine was kept. It was a brief but interplanetary journey. The hallway could've been in any office building anywhere—the drab carpet like an average of all color, the regulation Monets and mall pastels—but when I went through the double doors, there were the parents, stoic or chipper or haggard among flowers and balloons, and there were the children whose op notes I'd been typing, supine, surrounded by machines, their incisions covered lightly with gauze. Beneath the incisions, I knew, were the GORE-TEX patches newly anchored, the cusps of artificial valves opening and closing, the great vessels rerouted. I'd stir my coffee, averting my eyes, and drop my quarter in the slotted can.

The job was like that: I'd hammer away at descriptions of things I'd never seen, the bloodless words secreted by the green cursor, letter by letter, until the op note was done, and the patient had lived, and both Ross and I were dissolved into the note, his voice and my listening and the patient's revival distilled into the anonymity of Times 12. And then once in a while I could witness what I'd been writing about. I would visit the OR, I'd see a kid wheeled down the hall, I'd see parents in tears. I was always discovering what it was I'd been writing about, after the fact. I had described, but I had not seen.

"Think of it this way," said Bonnie, the nurse. "Suppose you're being attacked by a bear. A grizzly bear. Your body's going to send as much fluid as it can right into its tissues and keep it there for a while."

"So you don't bleed to death?" I asked.

"Right," she said. "Exactly. So when your daughter had her heart operated on, as far as she's concerned—that's like being attacked by a bear. Her body doesn't know the difference."

You could see it, looking at her face. She was puffy, her eyelids swollen. The catheter tube was nearly empty. Every hour the nurse would lift the tube, letting the urine run down to the graduated Lucite box. Eventually the doctors stepped up the diuretics. We had never been so happy to see urine. Tens of milliliters. Hundreds. The nurses smiling, the doctors smiling, everyone smiling. This was the beginning of recovery.

That night, Theresa's mom and Ellie came to the hospital to see Laura. They'd be flying back East the next morning, then returning in a week. We didn't know what Ellie would think, so we prepared her carefully, saying, "Now, we can't touch her, and she has a lot of tubes in her, and it might be a little scary . . ." But Ellie was used to seeing tubes by now. She walked in and said, "Hi, Laura!" Then she went over to the laptop and said, "Can I write something? Can I do e-mail?"

My mother-in-law, Carole, looked drawn but calm, sitting in the rocker. She'd felt as worried as Theresa or I, but she'd pushed it back for our sake. I think she was glad to see Laura with her own eyes.

Bonnie had been telling us about the camping trips she used to lead, the sing-alongs. I had my guitar and had been playing by Laura's bed. I knew it was a little ridiculous, the unconscious baby and the daddy playing heartfelt music to somehow get through to her, but I sang anyway. I'd started singing because Laura's blood pressure was high, and I thought the singing might calm her. One nurse had suggested it might: she'd seen the numbers change when parents came in the room. But mainly it was something for me to do, to make waiting easier.

So Bonnie and I sang. She stood at the wheeled desk, doing charts by a small reading light, her calm as focused as her daily talk was exuberant. We sang Ellie's favorite bedtime songs, "Angel from Montgomery," "Sweet Baby James," "Take Me Home, Country Roads," stopping now and then to remember the words. Next to me the ventilator drew the shapes of mechanical breath. Above me the flatscreen monitor shone like a campfire. Laura did not stir. In the opposite corner of the room were Theresa and Ellie, their faces lit by the laptop. As we sang, I had the guilty feeling that all this would be much worse if it were Ellie in the bed.

Medicine Is Communication

"Okay," said Ross, "let's pace her."

It was a couple of days after the operation. Laura was *in jet*, as the nurses said. *Jet* meant *junctional tachycardia*, which meant her heart was beating too fast. It ranged from the 180s to above 200. Even then I was losing my appetite for understanding exactly what this meant, and why it was happening. Her heart was beating too fast and that was bad and everyone wanted it to beat slower. I stood back and watched.

Ross picked up a gray box about the size of a Game Boy. It beeped when he turned it on. Then he picked up two wires that lay across the sheets, and plugged their exposed prongs into the box. At the other end of the wires was Laura's heart. There was a single blood-black stitch where each wire disappeared into the skin.

Ross twisted a knob, watching the monitor above Laura's head. The numbers didn't change. Behind him were the cardiac nurse, the other surgeon, the surgical PA, and the attending intensivist, all watching the monitor, in the respectful silence Ross tends to inspire. But the numbers stayed the same.

"Okay," he said, shrugging. "It was worth a shot. Let's keep an eye on her."

He turned to us. "Don't worry," he said. "Those numbers'll come down. She's going to be fine."

I remembered his absolute confidence from years ago. It's a good thing in a surgeon; you don't want someone picking up a scalpel above your infant daughter's anesthetized body, and then saying to himself,

Is this the right blade? Is this really what I want to be doing with my life, anyway?

June 19, 2001

Hi all-

No word on the website yet so I'll keep sending updates by email and clogging up your inboxes. George got some good sleep last night at our friends Matt and Judi's house as I took the night shift. Luckily, there were no more hypotensive episodes with Laura's blood pressure in the last 18 hours so that's good. However, Laura is starting to accumulate some fluid around her right lung (a pleural effusion) in addition to a bit of fluid in the lungs (pulmonary edema). This is curious because she's been on diuretics and peeing ALOT (~4cc/kg/hr, -750 ml over three days). They are going to insert a little drainage tube today and that will hopefully take care of the situation. Also, I suspect that she hasn't moved enough. I expect that we are in the ICU for a bit longer and in the hospital at least through the week. This is something of an unexpected setback for us. However, we are assured that this is not out of the ordinary in this situation.

As you might surmise, I've not been getting much work done here. However, I did watch a movie on the computer so I can now justify the expense :-) We've had a few visitors to lift our spirits. A good part of the day is spent talking with medical personnel and trying to understand jargon and changes in Laura's condition. I become mesmerized by all of the numbers on the monitors. Whenever the numbers change quickly, nurses and doctors come with speed, mutter acronyms, fiddle with dials, and then try to explain what happened. I suspect that when they mutter about PVCs, they are not talking about the plastic pipe in our bathroom.

I get exhausted by mid-afternoon each day from doing nothing but watching, waiting, and gathering information. It's a strange existence.

On other fronts, we understand that Ellie has taught herself to rollerblade while staying with Grandma and Aunt Susie.

Theresa

We spent about two weeks in the ICU, a week longer than we'd expected. There were complications, a secondary infection, fluid build-up around the lungs, oscillations in blood pressure, but even then we could see that Laura was, slowly, improving. Once they tried to let her breathe on her own, and she couldn't; then, two days later, she could, and she was extubated. She no longer needed the vent. We watched the numbers. We inspected the plastic bags on either side of the bed, looking at the fluid that had drained from her chest. We talked to Ellie, calling around until we found which of Theresa's sisters had her that day.

In the mornings the X-ray tech would wheel in the portable machine, I'd put on a lead apron, and they'd take another picture. I went with a nurse once to look at the morning's snapshot. She brought it up on a computer monitor in another room. Against the tracery of bone and lung and reclining heart, the intruding tubes were bright white: the NJ tube, threading the throat, coiled slackly in the stomach, its end in the jejunum; the pacer wires in the heart, the slim tubes in the right and left atria.

New nurses came on shift, new doctors, or nurses who'd been off since yesterday, since a few days ago, and we gave them the news. We told the story so far. Medicine is communication: the longer Laura had been in the hospital, the more her chart thickened—it looked like the Portland white pages before we left—the more her care depended on the oldest arts of human communication, the story basic to the tribe. Oral history. We became the keepers of our daughter's narrative; we changed it in real time, adding to it here, subtracting there, as the hours went by, the days. It was part of the central story of our family, the legend of who we had come to be.

It was a story we told, with variations, in daily e-mails to our friends. Since we'd found out, I'd been conjugating the fact: she has/had a heart defect, she will have/is having/has had surgery. We disconnected the room phone and plugged in the laptop. I unfolded Laura's recuperation like a serial novel, glancing from the flatscreen monitor on my lap to the one over my daughter's head. I adjusted the story for each person, editing out Laura's crashes for my mother, leaving out the lay explanations for Anjali and Nicole, both doctors. Each version was sonar, echolocation, the e-mails pinging the darkness outside the hospital room, our words coming back to us, transformed by distance.

And it may be that these repetitions, these rehearsals, helped me to understand the peculiar, underwater terrain of illness and parental love: that in navigating the dark, obstacle by obstacle, word by word, I managed, by accident, to constitute a landscape. It seems as likely that by telling stories, I sought not to comprehend the situation, but to avoid it. In the drained faces of friends, in the staticky pauses on the telephone, in the e-mail replies beginning *Re: Laura*, I saw that others understood the situation's core, the possible loss I had swathed in words. In their shocked responses to each medical update, I saw that I had transformed my life into a mere story, words drained of reference to the real, still-breathing daughter beside me. I knew it, and I liked it that way. I had anesthetized myself. I had reduced the story to an op note. Here I was, years later, with the same terminology, deadening the pain with toneless precision. I liked the nouns, the O_2 saturations, the mediastinal incisions; I liked the abbreviations, RA, LA, PA, the clipped medspeak of the ICU, the way it both conveyed the strangeness of our life, and kept that life at a distance. I avoided my life by facing it; I ignored the depths by describing the surfaces. Clearly I looked brave—I would rattle off fact after medical fact, and people would say, *how can you be so calm, I don't know how you manage it*—and really I was like the soldier whose leg is gone, his lucidity fueled by shock.

One night, when Laura seemed stable enough for us to go out, we left. We drove away from our unconscious daughter and went to a restaurant. We asked the nurses, is it okay? Can we both go out and eat? In another room on the unit, there was a girl, about two years old, who was unconscious and alone, day and night. There were whispers, an ugly breakup, parents living far away. But the nurses had smiled and sent us ahead. We ate at a restaurant that prides itself on its spicy food, its floor covered with peanut shells. On the walls were Polaroids of men who had eaten enough hot peppers to have their Polaroids taken.

We sat, freedom eclipsing guilt. We'd always left the hospital one at a time, the other keeping the vigil, and though our sense of urgency was fading, we were still at Care Level Six on the big white board by the ICU entrance. We'd come in at Level Seven. Seven was the night Laura crashed, and two cardiac nurses in the room, around the clock. Seven was the girl whose cancer had returned, and the young man whose pediatric heart defect had finally caught up with him, and the teenaged boy whose ATV had flipped, leaving him with multiple skull fractures. So it was good to be at Level Six. At Five we would leave for the newborn care unit, Laura suddenly enormous among the preemies, but for now we were still waiting.

Only by leaving the hospital, only by entering the miscellaneous world of shoppers and workers and children squalling in jogging strollers, could we glimpse what we were holding back. The hospital was beautiful, all that any parent could ask for. It had muted tile and stone and wood, and wide expanses of glass along the hallways, admitting what sunlight the Willamette Valley begrudges. The artwork was appropriately Northwestern, with the standard-issue mix of whimsy and reverence for nature that characterizes our summer festivals, the acrylically bright leaping salmon, the elk and beaver and turtles cast in bronze. It had a room for meditation, a quietly lit space with a radiating sun inlaid in the floor and a guest book filled with anguished prayers to Jesus. I felt lucky to be there, remembering the oppressive atmosphere of other hospitals I'd been in, the windowless hallways and cramped rooms, but in the end the effect was less healing than anesthetic. Inside the hospital, we were numb, separate. Deprived of comparison, we felt okay. Laura's blood pressure dropped then climbed, her infection responded to the third antibiotic they tried, and on and on, and we managed. We were fine. But when we emerged, the dream bubble burst. We'd smell air unscented by disinfectant, we'd walk on actual sidewalks, no one was wearing scrubs, there were no sobbing extended families spilling into the hallways, there were objects everywhere not individually wrapped for single use, and we felt like we'd won a dream vacation, an all-expenses-paid trip to the Disney World of normal life. It was kind of nice. We'd breathe in, deeply, and only then realize we'd been holding our breath.

We had one daughter watching *Cinderella* in Pennsylvania, and another in Intensive Care, but it was a date. When we got back to the hospital, we had to be buzzed back in, like teenagers after curfew. We went back upstairs. Everything was quiet. Laura was fine.

And then it was time to leave the ICU. Laura was breathing on her own, and her blood pressure was stable, though still high; so she was discharged to the Doernbecher Neonatal Care Center. The nurses called it the Dink.

It was strange to be leaving the ICU. We'd felt at home there, almost, the way a hotel room can come to seem almost yours. Our laundry spilled from a duffel bag, my guitar was propped in a corner, we'd taped Ellie's drawings to the wall. We ate takeout with chopsticks as Laura slept, glancing up at the heart monitor. Theresa pumped breast milk behind a privacy screen, labeling and dating and refrigerating each bottle; it all went sour in the end. Late at night I'd pad out to the break area in my socks and make espresso, with the gleaming machine a parent of transcendent understanding had donated to the unit. Though our room was as open as any stage to the central nurses' station, though our daughter's unsteady vitals were glowing in bright pastels above her head, and though, when we thought about it, we would rather be any-where else in the world, there was much about our stay in the ICU that was domestic and even sweet; and after a while there was no distin-guishing between our little rituals of belonging and the daily rituals of professional medical care, the X-rays, a change of diuretic, an adjust-ment of the ventilator setting, a swabbing of artificial tears into Laura's unconscious, half-open eyes. It was all part of the same effort, and on the best days, the sharp line between scrubs and street clothes blurred a little bit. We knew everyone by the time we left, and we liked most of the people we knew. We'd trusted them with our daughter's life, and they'd obliged us by saving her and keeping her well. At the same time, we knew we would probably never see any of them again.

So though we were overjoyed to be one step closer to the hospital exit, our departure from the ICU had an end-of-the-vacation feel to it. Theresa and Laura left first, the orderly pushing Laura's bed, and I stayed behind, shoving sweats and magazines and stray CDs into the duffel bag, unplugging the laptop from the phone jack, shutting the guitar in its case. The room felt bigger without the wheeled bed. The monitors were turned off, and the food and medicine pumps had been wheeled out to other rooms. Outside the weather had turned cloudy.

I got down to the Dink, where Laura was already installed, and from Theresa's face I could tell things were going poorly. There was one chair by the bed, and nowhere to put our things. The nurse looked about sixteen years old, sullen, passive, overworked. She didn't know where Laura's meds were. She didn't know where we could put our accumu-lated stuff. Every glance said we were in the way.

When we left, we had to sign out, then phone the desk clerks from the hallway to be let back in. The Dink was mainly for newborns, so security was tight. I noticed a memo posted by the telephone, with code words to say for different situations, ranging from "tense" to "violence imminent." Most of the babies were alone in their incubators. The ICU felt pure, tragic by comparison.

By nighttime Laura's medicines still hadn't arrived. Theresa had gone to a friend's house to get some rest. The high school–aged nurse had headed home, and in her place was a nurse I'll call Fred. Fred was a good nurse, attentive, calm, and competent, and around him I felt completely on edge. You meet people like that, human antitheses, pheromonal enemies. One sniff and everyone's hackles are up. We should've had plenty to talk about, what with him also being a nurturing male, but it didn't work that way. When I asked questions he was defensive; when I offered information, it seemed unwelcome. When I heard him telling another nurse Laura's blood pressure medication still hadn't arrived, I interrupted and said, "*What?* Her captopril *still* isn't here?" He rounded on me with a look just short of venomous. "It'll get here," he said. "I've already called twice."

At last he said, "Go ahead, get some sleep, we're fine here." In his voice, kindness outweighed irritation. He found me an unused room with a reclining chair and a thin hospital blanket. I thanked him and shut the door.

I couldn't sleep, so I began to write. I pushed the recliner aside, unfolded the laptop, lay down on the floor, and began a paragraph. I described the quiet of the Dink, the infants breathing, the machines breathing above them. The look of a backlit X-ray. I had written one poem since Laura's birth, a jagged draft rushed out in the days while we waited for the news of her diagnosis. The paper is coffee-stained; all the lines are crossed out. Since then, I'd written e-mails, a few journal entries, and the odd grocery list. But poetry was gone. It was a small strangeness eclipsed by the larger strangeness of having a daughter with

Down syndrome. I figured I might get back to poetry, maybe, someday. But at the same time, it seemed as if something more permanent had changed.

I tried not to think about what I was getting into. I thought I might have the beginnings of an essay. Even then I sensed the subject was too large for an essay or two, that a book was looming. On some level, it had been inevitable since Laura's arrival. Alone in the carpeted room, my daughter in an incubator next door, I remembered being nineteen, just beginning to write poetry. I didn't know what I was doing; I just knew I had to do it. In a relaxed moment the next day in the Dink, I told another nurse that I was writing about Laura. "Maybe you could send something to *Reader's Digest*," he said.

Strange to think of that time, at once accelerated and frozen, moment by moment. Of the decisions I made, easy as shrugging off a coat. I did not know I was trying to salvage, if not poetry, then the impulse behind it. To see if the tools of the old life might be adequate to the new.

On her last day in the hospital, Laura had an appointment with Anthony Wylie, a speech pathologist. Theresa had requested a consult on feeding techniques, and Anthony was coming to assess Laura and make recommendations. But since Theresa had a cold and couldn't be in the neonatal care center among the preemies, it was my job to listen and remember.

In the crowded hallway outside the unit, I talked with Theresa, pushing aside the habit of resentment, writing down the questions she wanted me to ask. I felt like a drunk suddenly wanting to focus, to show he can be sober.

I didn't want to. I just wanted to leave, deal with the feeding issues after we got home and settled in, at least get a little breathing space before we plunged right into the next campaign. Laura's heart was fixed. We were going home at last. One thing at a time. And yet I knew

Theresa was right to schedule the consult, and so, sitting by Laura's crib with Anthony, I watched him work with her. He was meticulous, circumspect, kind. I forced myself to watch closely, ask questions, write everything down. I was beginning to see what Theresa had already seen. The repair of Laura's heart—worried over endlessly, desperately—was only a beginning. Its closure was partial.

This is a difficult story to tell. Its high points are fleeting, not culminations, their timing inconvenient for drama, their significance misleading. They appear like random intrusions in a cliff wall. In the sedimentary accumulation of my life, I map the July Discontinuity. And finally, I have little accounting for the time, only an account. "Denial," Theresa was fond of saying then, "is a powerful coping tool." When I look back, I can hardly imagine what those people were going through.

It seems another life, and is, but it's more accurate to say that our lives stopped, then started again. For a long time I focused on the stopping part, the separation between then and now. In the end the continuities have proved more durable than the divisions. In this way, our family's story resembles the story of Laura's heart, which also had to be stopped, so she could go on.

I saw Ross once more before we left the hospital. I was downstairs in the deserted lobby, late at night, slumped in a soft chair. I looked up and saw him striding towards the front entrance. I called his name, and he turned. We talked briefly and I thanked him. "Sure," he said, turning to go. "Send me a picture sometime."

It occurred to me only later that, when Laura was in the hospital, I did not yet love her. I may only have been looking after her. Perhaps that was why, looking down at her prostrate in a hospital bed, I was glad she was not Ellie. Perhaps those early weeks were only a down payment on a love we might come to feel. Or I did not allow myself to love her, in order to save myself the pain.

Thinking this, I knew it was true; at the same time, I knew, because I *could* think it, it was no longer true.

I remember when the thought first occurred to me. It was August, some weeks after we'd gotten home from the hospital. I was in my workshop, holding Laura, in the ancient shed behind the house. I was looking for something essential to the furthering of a whim—a bolt, a tube of epoxy resin, an adjustable wrench, who knows what for who knows what project. Though I dislike football, and Guy is a dialect I speak only with difficulty, I do answer stress with power tools; I also look after children at home. So I held Laura, careful to keep her away from every sharp, pointed, and electrified thing in the shop, and rooted through sawdust and debris with my free hand.

She was braced in the crook of my left arm; I leaned away from her, to keep us both balanced. She twisted this way and that, inspecting the piles of offcuts from finished projects, the flickering shoplights, the exposed studs dark with age, the two-by-fours not "nominal," but actually two inches by four inches; and as I stood by the pull-down ladder, the late morning sunlight turning the dust over in its hands, I saw Laura, and realized what she was to me. I gathered her against me and told her so, in the best words I could find at the time. Then I carried her back into the house.

The Mayor of Hidden Valley

We came home from the hospital with six different medications, a cooler full of frozen breast milk, and a daughter with a newly repaired heart. It was late June. Laura was pink, breathing easily now, and though we were wary of infections, we knew she was on the mend.

But as an oral feeder, Laura had taken three giant steps back. Where she had simply refused to eat, she now resisted any approach to her mouth, with food, finger, or nipple. Anthony Wylie had given us an Infadent, which looked like an ear of rubber baby corn welded to a toothbrush handle. Its purpose was to accustom Laura to different textures, to having things in her mouth. She would suffer the Infadent to be touched to her lips; if it moved past her gums, or lingered on the center of her tongue, she would gag or throw up. This worsened in the first few weeks after we were home; one of her diuretics, it turned out, had nausea and vomiting as a side effect. When we were allowed to take her off the diuretic, the vomiting stopped, but the instinctive gagging remained.

What Laura was experiencing is called "oral aversion." When children receive trauma to the mouth and airway, they shut down. Given a choice between food and air, they choose air. And Laura had had trauma in spades. She'd had the nose tube, which was not only unpleasant in itself—adults describe it as a disagreeable tickle in the back of the throat—but was also associated with the experiences of her first hospitalization, including oxygen deprivation, twenty or so needlesticks, the act of taking the nose tube in and out, adhesive tape allergies, and the respiratory illness itself. All this, of course, was minor in comparison to the more recent trauma of surgery and recuperation. How much of this Laura had been aware of, and what "awareness" might mean for a three-month-old infant under heavy sedation, is unclear; what is clear is that when she came home from the hospital, her aversion to anything approaching her mouth had greatly increased. In time, the gagging faded somewhat, but she showed no signs of hunger. Thanks to the nose tube, she wasn't hungry anyway. Her belly filled, reliably, on clock time, day and night.

For the rest of the summer, we simply kept on. We saw specialists. We stimulated Laura's gums with the Infadent during pump feeds to help her associate oral activity with eating. We tried one new nipple after another, translucent caricatures of the breast. We tried sippy cups, Avent cups, cutout cups, cups with long spouts, short spouts, flow regulators—plastic chalices, ceremonial vessels for the rite of medical nutrition, but Laura was an unwilling convert. She flinched and turned away.

Each night, Theresa tried nursing her. Laura would latch on happily and play; as soon as the milk reached the back of her throat, she'd gag. Once she shocked us by nursing well for twenty minutes, late at night in the big wooden rocker. She never did this again, though we tried to duplicate the conditions. Still, Theresa kept pumping breast milk, losing sleep, a steady effort despite eroding hopes. Another day, determined to simply *move past* Laura's aversion, I got an entire ounce of water into her by syringe, squirting in two-tenths of a milliliter at a time; if she got more than that, she choked and gagged. I cuddled her, smiling, laughing, saying, Yay Good Job Hooray Hooray, thinking *eat, dammit, eat,* and the next day, I couldn't get a drop into her. She cried, shut her lips, and turned her head from the syringe.

She still needed nourishment. She still, evidently, experienced a kind of hunger: fussy before a pump feed, she was calm afterwards. But she did not associate these sensations with eating. What she had lost was *appetite,* the neurological link between pleasure and satiety. We

felt as if an absolute limit had been reached. We could have ghostly pictures taken of our daughter's heart, have her anesthetized and cut open
and repaired, we could read *People* in the surgical waiting room, both
terrified and calm, but despite our best efforts as parents, we could not
make Laura *want* to eat. As the summer dragged on, day by beautiful
Northwestern day, we celebrated what tiny progress we saw, and we
worried whether it would be enough. The nose tube was not an indefinite solution. Already the developmental pediatrician in Portland had
recommended surgical placement of a gastrostomy tube, which would
bypass the esophagus, providing a port in her belly. If she never learned
to eat by mouth, we could still pump food into the port.

Facing the prospect of a G tube, I began to understand what Theresa
had been through, over the NG tube. I saw what she had seen, or fore-
seen—that accurate unease, not anxiety, but intuition—and understood, too, the loneliness of it, of having that intuition scanted or dis-
missed. Feeding Laura was still personal for Theresa, in a way it could
not be for me. It was her issue, and always had been. But it had become
our issue too.

It was late August, and Ellie was seething for kindergarten to start. She
went to Safety Town, a pre-K day camp, where the children learned
about traffic safety, animal safety, bus safety, pool safety, and bad strangers. There were songs for each kind of safety. An entire model town was
set up on the gymnasium floor, a tarpaulin printed with streets and
crosswalks, scaled-down buildings, a church, a school, a courthouse.
There were kid-sized pedal-operated cars. You had to pause and look
both ways, crossing the pretend streets. I was in heaven. Since February
Laura had been in and out of hospitals, and here was a model town
devoted entirely to not being hurt. When I dropped Ellie off there,
my heart filled with a security half resembling joy. At home Ellie ran
through the house, singing STOP LOOK AND LISTEN, colliding with
walls on purpose and falling down. How many days, Dad? How many

days till school starts? I can't WAIT! And she'd run off laughing.

Her first full day of kindergarten was September eleventh. I woke up and logged on to the Net and read that a plane had crashed into the Twin Towers. No details. Theresa was sitting in the big chair, trying to get Laura to nurse; I said to turn on the TV. A few minutes later the South Tower collapsed. The rectangle in the corner of the screen said LIVE. It was happening, it had already happened. Ellie didn't register the event. She was frantically organizing her backpack for school.

By early September, we'd begun to feel stalemated. We'd switched away from Anthony Wylie, the hospital speech therapist, to a feeding clinic—a team of specialists—and we were beginning to regret the switch. The clinic seemed to have run out of ideas. The goal was still bottle-feeding or nursing, Laura wasn't bottle-feeding or nursing, and there were no more cups or nipples to try.

One morning in mid-September, Theresa took Laura down to a new feeding clinic in Eugene. It was closer than Portland; we had nothing to lose. When Theresa came back from Eugene, she said, "Laura ate eight ounces by mouth."

"You lie," I said. "No way."

"Yes way," she said. "She ate Cheez Whiz."

A sunny day, new flags blowing everywhere, flags in shop windows and car dealerships, flags downloaded, printed, and taped in the rear windows of minivans. We drove to Wendy's for lunch. I interrogated Theresa, asking questions through my half-chewed double cheese no mayo no mustard, happy, reminding myself not to be happy.

If you counted actual quantities, Theresa explained, Laura had probably eaten closer to four ounces. Much had been spit out, dribbled out, or batted away. Laura had struggled and cried; she had literally choked down her lunch, which had also included pudding, cream cheese, and part of a graham cracker.

Every good day in memory seemed sunny and windy: Ellie's birth,

Laura's birth, the day we visited the Eugene branch of the Children's Development and Rehabilitation Center. I watched the traffic out on Ninth Street and sipped my Coke, pursing my lips, forming the vacuum, controlling the rate of flow. I was not surprised by the bubbles. I did not fear the liquid approaching the back of my throat.

When Theresa described the clinic, she was happier than I'd seen her in some time. She'd liked the people. They listened. They were thorough. They'd been organized: they were on time, they had a tray of food ready. They were informed: they'd actually read the chart, and they knew Laura's medical history in detail, mentioning things even we had forgotten. They even knew I was an at-home dad. This mattered to them because a child eats in a social context. To feed the child, you have to understand the child's family. As a more practical matter, you need to know who's doing feeding therapy during the day. The clinicians also worked well as a team. They deferred to each other easily and without ego. If they disagreed, they worked together towards a composite answer.

When they examined Laura, they decided two things right away. One was that she would eat again, that she had both the muscles and the oral skills to "organize" food and swallow. The other was that there was no longer any point in trying to get her to nurse or take a bottle. It had been four months since she last nursed, not counting the one time in the rocking chair. So it was on to solid food.

The question was: Why Cheez Whiz?

They were pro–wheat bread, in general, so they'd been a little embarrassed about it. But Cheez Whiz was an ideal baby food for Laura. It was sticky, which made it hard to spit out, essentially forcing her to swallow. It was also high in calories, an advantage for children whose oral consumption is measured in milliliters. And most of all, it had a strong taste, appropriate for the unsubtle palate of a six-month-old. Sweet, salty, sour, bitter: the idea was to combat aversion with pleasure, to pit the palate against the gag.

There was specific behavioral advice to follow, as well. Use different-colored spoons, for one, so that she would not focus on one object and associate it with the unpleasantness of eating. Hide the spoon between bites. Use a toy to distract her: they had a windup toy that unreeled a Mickey Mouse animation, which she watched with fascination, less conscious of the food in her mouth, the threat of choking. If she gags, don't overreact. Tip her head forward and speak in a soothing voice. Have her eat with you, when you eat. Pull her high chair up to the table. Use the nose tube for supplemental nutrition, but don't feed her while the pump is running. In other words, begin teaching her the meaning of food; it may be Cheez Whiz, but she is still breaking bread.

Their approach contrasted sharply with that of the nutritionist we'd met back in May. They were clearly more experienced, more knowledgeable about Down syndrome and eating problems, but the real difference was philosophical. They saw Laura not only as a member of a category—a child with feeding problems—but also as a *person*, an individual with emotions and instincts and preferences. This insight was central, not incidental, to their recommendations.

It's good to feel hopeful, even in a Wendy's. It had been a long half year. Most of what we had felt was simply new: we had no precedent for Down syndrome, heart surgery, feeding problems, or for the tense separations that followed in their wake, the daily fissures in our voices. This was, for a change, familiar. It felt good.

Theresa and I have been together for over twenty years, and have consumed an embarrassing number of square beef patties in that time. Our consumption of fast food divided us from many of our friends, especially the ones who used to go with us for late night triple cheeseburgers, then later became vegetarians, then had kids and started eating meat again. In their vegetarian years, the burgers were a secret shame. Our own habit dates mainly from the cross-country driving trip we took after college, our grand tour of cities and National Parks and kitsch. We began in high hopes of sampling inexpensive regional cuisine, hopes that ended with stomach cramps in a tent somewhere in the Arizona desert. Aversion is aversion: as we've found with Laura, the logic of nausea and vomiting is absolute. We chose mediocrity over charm. Besides, the mediocrity was air-conditioned. We were driving in a 1974 Toyota Corolla with no AC and an engine sized for a riding mower, and after hours of slowly unreeling prairie or desert in what was basically a convection oven with wheels, we came to depend on the shockwave of refrigerated air scented with deep-fry oil. It was a powerful reinforcement. We might not discover the world's greatest unknown pecan pie, but we wouldn't get food poisoning either, and we could at least cool off and sit for a while.

Anyway, the trip wasn't about the food. It was a six-week audition for the future, a tour of the country we might live in together. It was promising, though no promises were made; and it's good, now, to look back and see that the flashes of hope I felt were glints of something durable, sustaining, true to a future that happened, if not exactly as we expected. For better or worse, I still associate our hopeful beginnings with swan-necked ketchup dispensers, disposable straws, melamine tables, waxy yellow cups beaded with condensation, and portraits of a still-living Dave Thomas. It felt perfectly normal to be sitting in a tinted-glass atrium, eating wilted French fries, and feeling as if things might work out.

So we began the next phase of teaching our daughter to eat. Predictably, her success before the gathered clinicians was atypical, a statistical outlier. At home, she proved more recalcitrant. She gagged and spat and cried. She got down maybe a tenth of what we put in her mouth. But it felt, to us, like a real start.

October 2001

I assemble my materials: Cheez Whiz, Nutella, guacamole prepared with mayonnaise, 24 cal./oz. formula, flavored cream cheese, bean dip, pudding, Laura, washcloth, tablespoon, flat spoon, Infadent, cutout cup, plasticized bib (large), high chair with tray, plate, pad and pencil, dog. I strap Laura in the high chair, fasten the bib, and turn on the TV. She'll gain weight like any other American: eating junk food, watching cable, her consciousness of taste and texture diluted by image and sound.

The towers collapse on every channel, unthinkable and unavoidable. I switch to the Teletubbies: PBS is keeping its children's programming terrorism-free. I pick up the Infadent and turn towards Laura. Behind me, a bunch of color-coded, adult-sized bionic infants are conversing in their human bird language, an indistinct group chirping that sways from celebration to dismay. Oh-oh! Oh-oh! They have video monitors in their abdomens, they live in a miniature golf course, and their deity is a laughing infant who rises like the sun. I remember the anecdote I heard in an undergraduate poetry workshop: a French poet visited America, saw Bugs Bunny for the first time, and pronounced a surrealist poem impossible here. The country was already surreal.

I begin with the Infadent, tapping it to Laura's lips. I let her play with it, chewing and sucking. This is the equivalent of stretching before a run. Eating is an athletic event: muscles are used, calories are expended. I am "waking up the mouth muscles." Next, I massage Laura's cheeks with index finger and thumb, beginning at the cheekbones and moving towards the mouth, using moderate pressure. I try to be gentle but definite. So far so good.

I open the jar of Cheez Whiz and dig out one tablespoon. It is a difficult substance to measure—it sticks to everything, which is the point—but I do my best, and scrape it off onto the plate. It looks daunting, enormous. It is also unmelted, which is the wrong consistency for Cheez Whiz. When we lived in Philadelphia and Theresa was finishing her doctorate at Penn, we used to go to Abner's for cheesesteaks; Theresa got Provolone, I got Cheez Whiz. (One of the postdocs in Theresa's doctoral lab occasionally drew blood from student volunteers, which he purified for experiments. When he centrifuged the blood, he said he could tell, from the thin yellow meniscus in the test tube, when the donor had eaten a cheesesteak for lunch.)

I take the flat spoon, carve out a yellow glob, and present it to Laura's lips. She presses her lips together. I nudge her lips with the spoon; she refuses to open up. I turn up the TV volume. I make faces. I jump up and down. Finally I push the spoon past her lips. It's a fine line between therapy and aggression, a line we've walked for weeks, and as multiple scars attest, love has resembled violence for quite a while now. Laura looks surprised, betrayed. She works her cheeks and jaw, trying to maneuver the Cheez Whiz away from her throat. She can't do it, and she begins to gag: coughing, flinching, her eyes wide open, beginning to tear up. I try not to overreact. I tip her head forward, make encouraging noises, let her work through it. I am trusting the therapists, who told me she wouldn't asphyxiate. I am depending on the very oral aversion I'm trying to combat: her hyperdeveloped gag reflex will protect her.

I give her a rest. I try the other foods, in smaller quantities. I record the quantities. I try cup drinking, which is a total failure. All the while Penny is sitting at the base of the high chair, in the desperately attentive posture of a good student hoping to be noticed. When fragments fall, she immediately wolfs them down. Penny has ballooned in size over the years: she began as a whippet-thin rescue, but with Ellie, and now Laura, dropping food from high chairs, she began her steady march up the veterinarian's wall chart, from Dog 1 (emaciated) to Dog 5 (morbidly obese). Penny is well into Dog 4.

The Teletubbies are done with whatever they were chirping about, so I shut the TV off. Breakfast is over. I untie the bib, lift Laura from the high chair, waltz her around the living room, comforting, telling her good job, good job. I am trying to associate positive experiences with eating. I am apologizing too.

— ◆ —

In late October, we visited the Eugene clinic again. Though the six weeks had seemed equivocal, filled with failure, Christine Jepsen, the RN in charge of the clinic, felt we'd made real progress. So did Jan Lee, the physical therapist: "Like night and day," she said, shaking her head. We'd seen it, sort of, but for them, Laura was a flower blooming in time-lapse.

Now three problems remained:

1. Laura tolerated food, but didn't particularly like it. She had oral skills, but not appetite.

2. She tolerated liquids least of all, but she needed liquids most of all: about sixteen ounces of formula per day.

3. The nose tube had been in a really long time; it wasn't clear how much longer we could avoid the gastrostomy tube.

So the gagging was reduced, and Laura could swallow. We still needed her to *want* food. And even if she turned out to like, say, Cheez Whiz, it wasn't what she needed: she had to want formula. Ideally, this would happen soon enough to avoid stomach surgery. The feeding team said—cautiously—that as long as Laura was making progress, and as long as the nose tube didn't seem to be doing harm, we could leave it in for another six weeks. The pediatric gastroenterologist, whom we saw a few days later, concurred. We had a stay.

To heal Laura, to get her to eat, we would have to provoke her appetite. So we did what we'd been doing since we'd switched to solid foods: we shopped. I went into supermarkets, plunked Laura's car seat in the middle of the cart, and went down one aisle, then the next, scanning from top to bottom. Anything that looked promising went in the cart. I wanted fat; I wanted calories. A tide of cans and packages rose slowly around the car seat: Reddi-Wip, aerosolized spray cheese, cream cheese in salmon, strawberry, and jalapeno flavors, cherry pie filling, smoked oysters, chocolate chip cookie dough, ready-made cake icing in chocolate, vanilla, and butterscotch, Bosco, strawberry Quik, Quaker

Instant Oatmeal (variety pack), cream of mushroom soup, cream of chicken soup, New England clam chowder, Manhattan clam chowder, bean with bacon soup, canned turkey gravy, Ben and Jerry's, Häagen-Dazs, Breyers, Dreyer's, Thousand Island dressing, and drinkable yogurt. Laura looked around, surrounded by cans. She was like a reverse cornucopia: we were trying to stuff the food *in*. She sat placidly in the midst of plenty.

In the supermarket, I saw with a paradoxical eye: I was foraging and impulse shopping at once. I turned aside the bright graphics on each can, favoring the black-and-white text of nutritional fact. But what I was seeking was precisely what the images promised: the one taste whose joy would overwhelm her, and make her want more.

As it turned out, ranch dressing was the key to everything. Without ranch dressing, my daughter would have a port in her stomach.

We discovered this partly through trial and error, and partly through systematic observation. We'd long ago figured out that Laura didn't have much of a sweet tooth. You'd think any child would cry hallelujah on being asked to eat Nutella all day, but Laura liked salmon-flavored cream cheese better. In my ramblings through the supermarket, moving from label to FDA-required label, I'd discovered that salad dressings were incredibly calorie-rich, and ranch dressing was richest of all. If you got one ounce into her, that was one hundred and twenty calories, the same as six ounces of formula. That November, on my thirty-seventh birthday, as we sat with a few friends in the sleepy haze of a fading sugar rush, we tried ranch dressing on Laura. Our friend Robert lifted a tiny spoonful to her mouth. She tasted it and thought for a minute. Then her mouth gaped open for more.

It was a lucky moment, a moment when we see the latent become visible, the inactive activated. She wanted food, so she opened her mouth. When the food was in her mouth, she knew what to do: she could "organize" it, shunt it back towards her throat, and swallow. She had no evident fear of choking, or of losing air. After she swallowed, she opened her mouth, to show us she wanted more. It was communication, exchange. I squeezed out more ranch dressing onto the spoon.

It was good news; in retrospect, it was the turning point. But it wasn't enough.

She still needed formula. When Leslie Houghton, the feeding team's nutritionist, had insisted on sixteen ounces of formula per day, Theresa and I had resisted. It seemed a huge amount. And why formula, I wanted to know. Why couldn't she get all of her calories from Hidden Valley Ranch Dressing? Why couldn't we just make up the difference with liquid vitamins? Wasn't there some kind of astronaut food we could get hold of? I kept these objections to myself. The answer was simple: lacking breast milk—in the name of sanity and sleep, Theresa had stopped pumping—formula was the best option we had. It took Laura's nutritional needs into account in a way ranch dressing did not. The fact that Laura disliked it was irrelevant.

I'd been working on the formula problem for some time. I'd already tried using other liquids to reconstitute formula powder, like pineapple juice. ("You might want to try that yourself," Christine had said, "before you give it to her.") I'd also mixed formula with mayonnaise and avocado, made formula banana smoothies, and pulverized any number of foods in the Happy Baby Food Grinder, mixing formula into the orange paste of SpaghettiO's, the brown paste of beef stew, the colored flecks of mixed vegetables. These had been accepted, more or less, but not enjoyed. I'd mixed strawberry syrup and Bosco into formula, and I'd reconstituted milk-based soups with formula in a one-to-one ratio: cream of mushroom, celery, chicken, and New England Clam Chowder. No luck.

I began cooking with formula. I made formula tapioca and formula alfredo. I went through the supermarket and found the Knorr sauce mix display and took one packet of each: Hollandaise, white, four cheeses, and "seafood." This was still before the ranch dressing break-through, the junk food eureka, and when I think of the things I stuffed into her, I'm amazed I didn't seal her lips for good.

Part of the problem with formula was taste, but part was texture. Laura could not "organize" thin liquids: they evidently distressed her in the way they rushed towards the back of her throat. Gloria Wong, the occupational therapist, had shown me the trick of thickening for-mula with rice cereal, so Laura could handle the texture. So I thickened the formula, sprinkled Hidden Valley Powdered Ranch Dressing Mix on top, and offered a spoonful of the mixture to Laura. She ate it like a baby bird.

I told Theresa, "I am the mayor of Hidden Valley."

We had three weeks until our next clinic appointment. We kept on feeding Laura her flavored, thickened formula; we charted her daily intake, tablespoon by tablespoon. In the second week of November, the nose tube came out by accident, and we decided to leave it out. Soon after, we returned the infusion pump. As the meaning of appetite be-gan to dawn on Laura, the connections between pleasure and variety and fullness, she began to eat foods she had originally rejected: cream of mushroom soup, stew, gravy. In December, we handed a stained yel-low pad to Leslie Houghton, the handwritten columns headed Ounces Formula and Ounces Total, and after a long time with pencil and cal-culator, she decided Laura's intakes would be sufficient. At that clinic visit, we began discussing how to undo the foundation of what we'd done: to get Laura on a moderate-calorie diet, to begin thinning her formula, so she could drink it straight. Six weeks later, in February, we got the go-ahead to forget about formula, and start on whole milk. We talked about "grading," or opening the mouth to the appropriate size; Laura still gaped wide at a cup, when she only needed to open her mouth a fraction. Jan Lee, the physical therapist, suggested a light pres-sure beneath Laura's chin. It was then I knew the house of feeding was built, and we were hanging a wreath on the door. At the end of the visit, Christine said Laura had graduated and didn't need to come back.

Soon Laura was eating everything put in front of her. Our second daughter is nothing if not decisive. She'd take a bottle easily, draining it by ounces, as if nothing had ever been wrong. We watched the tiny bubbles coursing upwards. We watched like desert travelers, fooled too often by mirages, unwilling to believe that the oasis is real.

We were relieved, unspeakably relieved, and yet what did our experience tell us about Laura's future? Would everything take this much work? Would we always speak Medical English, part jargon, part ordinary speech? An occupational therapist observes Laura chewing, moving food from one side of her mouth to the other, and says, "Oh, what beautiful lateralization!" A surgeon says, "Yeah, we'll just ligate that off when we're in there." We had learned that language too, and found ourselves speaking it without thinking. We had been living in the light of science, and in that bright light every word had a second shadow. Every savory word, *butter, sugar, rice*, was shadowed by the dry and tasteless vocabulary of calories, milliliters, and syringes. Nourishment was shadowed by nutrition.

That year, in my bitterest moments—*bitterness* being the taste of poison, the evolved displeasure that says, Do Not Eat—I'd think, Great. Another climb out of the canyon, just to get to the plateau where other children are already toddling towards the horizon, hand in hand with happy parents. Our frustrations with eating became a species of a general discontent: the longing, wistful and bitter by turns, for the normal childhood, the one that was supposed to happen. It is, of course, nostalgia for a projection. It dies hard. Even now, years later, it feels sometimes as if the rest of the world is light enough to walk on clouds and live in cities there, while we have sunk, under the weight of a single chromosome, into a valley of intermittent rain.

I don't know if I'd feel any different with another child. I doubt it. A mild but real depression has accompanied me for as long as I can remember. In her six-year-old way, Ellie knew this, and knew to give me room when she saw a bleak stare cross my face, or when she heard kitchen drawers slamming. I had raised her at home while Theresa worked, and so she had become, like Theresa, a scholar of my moods. And like Theresa, she was circumspect enough, even then, to absolve me with pharmacology. Looking up from her after-school bowl of Rice Krispies, she'd say: "Dad. You need a cup of coffee." This helped. So did even a minute spent with Laura, who was learning to clap her hands, and who was, to our delight, beginning to recognize us: at the dinner table, as she sat above the mess on her high chair tray, we'd ask, "Where's Mum-mum? Where's Da-Da? Where's Ellie?" She'd turn, dependably, towards each, as we were named.

To eat is to taste belonging. For me, growing up, it was sticky rice, on the table virtually every night. I poured soy sauce over it, because I liked the taste, and every night my mother shook her head. It was a double insult. She had known starvation during the war, so to treat food this way was wrong. And besides, you just didn't put soy sauce on rice. I was a spoiled American, pouring on the soy sauce because I liked it that way. Now, when my mom visits, Ellie puts soy sauce on her rice too, shy but defiant.

Beneath the specifics—soy sauce, rice, Hidden Valley Ranch Dressing powder—lie the stories: not only the family stories, but the biochemical story, the body guided by a tongue to the molecules it needs, and the developmental story too. In eating, the mouth prepares for speech.

As Laura's first birthday approached, as she made it through colds without hospitalization, and then, miraculously, began to feed herself, I realized that what I really wanted was a celebration. I wanted to throw a party. We would invite everyone the house could hold.

For a year we had withdrawn. It was only one paradox in a newly paradoxical life: we were suddenly closer to our friends, they'd helped us in a thousand ways, and yet we'd turned inward, tracing a circle around ourselves. The birthday party would open the circle. It would ratify a turning point, a shift from the medical to the social, an official debut in the community. A return to normal. I had lots of ideas about what it would mean, but Theresa just thought it would be fun to have a party.

She brushed out the wispy bird's nest of Laura's hair, clipped in a barrette, and dressed her in velvet. I made jambalaya and rice. About forty people came, counting the kids. Matt and Judi came with Maris, and Jami and Garvin came with Zel and Tessa—two families driven north to Portland, looking for better jobs, a better constellation of home and work. It's a contradiction particularly evident in this town: among all the trappings of rootedness, people are always moving away.

But for now there was homemade bread, salsa from the co-op, salads strewn with edible flowers, cakes, pints of ice cream. Beer, wine, tequila. We'd said no presents were necessary, a wish genially ignored, and there were as many presents for Ellie as for Laura. Ellie was told, over and over again, what was and is true: what a good big sister she'd been, and how lucky Laura was. Some friends had pitched in and gotten us a night out, a gift certificate at a local restaurant, money for a sitter. We said, "Oh, you shouldn't have," and they smiled sweetly and said, "Whatever."

The kids ran, screamed, and played Pin the Nose on the Nutritionist. Theresa had commissioned a sketch, and Robert had shown up with a large charcoal sketch of a doleful woman, eyes downcast. Theresa hung it on the wall. Then she took Laura's nose tube, scissored it into pieces, and stuck strips of tape on the pieces. The kids lined up, and we blindfolded them and steered them towards the cardboard, each one waggling the yellow bit of #5 nasal-gastric tube. The model for the nutritionist, we later found out, was the painting of Mary in the Sistine Chapel.

Stacy and Johnson came down from Portland, bringing Elijah; we'd met them during Laura's first hospitalization. Elijah and Laura sat next to each other on a blanket. It was good to see them there together: Elijah with his café au lait skin and dark looping curls, Laura with her indescribable eye color, her sparse flat hair. Watching them, I hoped that Laura would find friends and equals, and that she would attain independence, yet not be alone. We've often wondered if living in a city, and not a college town of fifty thousand, might not give Laura advantages: there'd be more choices in adapted recreation, more people with Down syndrome to make friends with. When high school arrives, when the hormone-fueled sexual economy ramps up, when Laura begins to collide with world history and trigonometry—then, I think, the question of belonging, of who Laura's peers are, will become more urgent.

We were gossiping about cardiologists, trading updates on tubes and medications. Occasionally I noticed a glance our way, someone hesitating, then deciding not to join in. We sat on the floor, Stacy, Johnson, Theresa, and me, and inside the circle we made were our two children with Down syndrome, the warmth of shared experience, the sense of a restored future. I felt an invisible border of definition, tightening around us. Outside it were conversations about weaning, sleeping through the night, and jobs in California. A conga line of preschoolers careened in from the kitchen, followed by laughter and calls to slow down.

That April, Laura returned to the hospital. She'd had a low-level cold for weeks, but then it worsened, into lethargy and fever. She drowsed against me all day, against Theresa all night, and cried feebly, pitifully, if we tried to set her down. Her breathing rattled and caught on phlegm. We ran the humidifier, or filled the bathroom with steam, and nothing changed. And she stopped eating. We brought out the current favorites: plain boiled rice, Saltines, canned mandarin oranges. I even fixed rice cereal with formula and ranch dressing, already a Golden Oldie on the nutritional jukebox, but she cried and turned away. Soon we were counting orange segments consumed and syringing drops of water into her mouth. She all but refused her blood pressure medication, and when we tried to give her liquid Tylenol, her face contorted and reddened, her back arched, and her hand batted the dropper away. When we'd gotten the pink syrup in her mouth, she spat it back out. Her lips were dry, her diapers light, with a trace of amber urine: she was beginning to dehydrate. We decided to have her admitted.

She had pneumonia. It was one year, almost to the day, since her first hospitalization. Then, too, a bad cold had spiraled downward. We braced ourselves against fear. Not so much, this time, the sickening, vertiginous fall: it was more like a dull familiarity, a sense of an inescapable fate. We put it all aside. We called friends to watch Ellie and walk Penny. Theresa called work and said she wouldn't be in. We were old hands now, used to the supercaffeinated sense of purpose, the checklist for setting a life aside, the trick candle of fear.

But at fourteen months, with a repaired heart, Laura was far sturdier than the nine-week-old infant we'd once rushed to the ER. There was no ambulance to Portland. Her IV went in easily, without the screaming, oxygen-depriving ordeals of the year before. There was no NG tube. Dr. E., who'd broken the news to us about Laura's Down syndrome, oversaw Laura's care; his affection for her, his familiar presence, and his clear discussion of medical options made the experience tolerable. Laura's fever came down, and she came home after two days.

For a few weeks afterwards, I made everyone wash their hands as soon as they came in the house. But after a while I let it go. Even I could tell Laura was going to be fine.

At Home

To write a book about a child with Down syndrome, as that child grows, is to understand that life is water. It runs, slips, evaporates, changes course, and what seems an eternal truth—a child on a ventilator, a child who won't eat, a child who hasn't spoken—evaporates, leaving a changing present. Already Laura's heart surgery felt long ago; she still took her heart medicine, and we still went to the weird-smelling compounding pharmacy to get it. But cardiology was a footnote now, not the main story. So the story I had to tell was changing too.

For a year, I had felt like a parent to one child, and a triage nurse to another. In the shock of diagnosis, I saw only the differences between them: the perforated heart, the changed brain, the slack muscle tone, the extra chromosome. And yet these facts were as deceptive as they were verifiably true. The differences were real, but their meaning was less fateful than I had supposed. This was true, I was learning, not only for hearts and brains, but for chromosomes as well.

Until then, I'd contented myself with a simple understanding of molecular genetics: Laura had one extra chromosome, which caused all the damn trouble. This was convenient, for a writer. It was easier to riff on chromosomes if you didn't actually know what they did. But it was becoming clear to me that making metaphors from chromosomes, without at least a rudimentary understanding of how they worked, might not be without its problems. That understanding a genetic disorder might mean understanding something about genes.

I began to look things up and to talk about what I had learned, which produced the smile Theresa gets when I try to talk about science.

"It's not," she said, "as simple as having one extra chromosome. It's that there's more protein, overexpressed."

She explained: a chromosome is not a *thing*, a mysterious totemic object. It's a set of directions for producing proteins. Without these directions, no fertilized egg could develop into a child, and no child could live: the complex miracle of embryology, and the ordinary miracle of maintaining cell pH, and everything in between, are modulated by proteins, synthesized in the proper quantities, and at the proper time. Since Laura had one more twenty-first chromosome than most other people, each of her cells had, in effect, a surfeit of directions: the proteins are "overexpressed." This had not only affected her embryonic development, but continues to affect her in the present.

The more I learned about the forty-seventh chromosome, the less it lent itself to metaphor. I'd compared the chromosome to a black mark, the missing apostrophe in Down syndrome, the weight that pulled us away from other parents. These metaphors, though true to the way I felt, had their limitations. First, they treated the chromosome as static and singular, rather than dynamic and multiple; in so doing, I ignored the chromosome's *function*, its connection to the past of the species, and its role in the daily work of the body. Second, by isolating the chromosome as "extra," I reinforced Laura's separation from other, bisomic children. Third, I allowed myself to trace all our troubles to a single, biological cause.

I had seen my lyrical sentences as a way of resisting an impersonal diagnosis, and of witnessing to Laura's true dignity as a human being. It had not occurred to me that my metaphors might be complicit in everything I was trying to combat.

I was learning, again, the lesson I'd been learning all year: as a father and a writer, I would need to avoid the dead ends, the red herrings, the patterns both obvious and false. It had been true with the extraordinary but insignificant coincidence of meeting Ross Ungerleider again, and it was true in considering my second daughter's genetic makeup.

For a poet, one imaginatively productive falsehood is worth a dozen dry accuracies. But I wasn't writing poetry anymore.

It's clear, in retrospect, that I had things precisely backwards. I'd thought I was beginning with biological fact and writing my way towards an understanding of my daughter. Rather, I'd begun, unwitting, with a social understanding, which had driven my understanding of biological fact. I had begun by assuming that Laura was essentially different from me. Because I believed this, I had isolated the heart, the chromosome, the eyes, and focused on what was different about them. In doing so, I had failed to see what she and I shared.

Just before Laura's hospitalization, we had met with her therapists to discuss her progress and to set goals for the coming year; and of the seven areas of concern enumerated in Laura's Individual Family Service Plan—Cognitive, Adaptive, Social or Emotional, Physical (Gross Motor), Physical (Fine Motor), Communication (Receptive), and Communication (Expressive)—it was the last that mattered to us most. To speak clearly is to have a chance, at least, at belonging.

Speech, like eating, is as complex as it is ordinary. With typically developing children, the complexities are obscured. When Ellie began to talk—she said her first word, *light*, on an airplane, pointing up at the reading lamp—we were surprised and happy. But we hadn't talked to a speech pathologist, and we didn't know that her tongue had to be behind her upper teeth to pronounce the *l*. She was eight months old. Laura, at fifteen months, seemed stalled. She could say *da da da*, and that was it. In a no-stone-unturned sort of way, we consulted a private speech pathologist, who told us, airily, that the syllable *zh* was "years away," and that children with Down syndrome often call Mom *Bob*, having difficulty with *m*.

We decided to alter our approach. For now, Communication (Expressive) would mean not speech, but Sign.

We had been signing at Laura almost since birth. We had dutifully followed the advice Pat Hill gave us: Limit yourself to a few signs, do them consistently, and say the word as you do the sign. We stuck with *more*, which seemed a natural for any child. The private speech pathologist had commented that she thought it was too "abstract." Abstract or not, it resonated with us. What could be more obvious to a child than *more*? What's more palpable than absence? *More* is performed by gathering fingertips to thumbs of each hand, then tapping the gathered fingertips together. From the front, the sign looks like a gate opening and closing.

Throughout the spring, I opened and closed the gate above Laura's high chair. Above spoonfuls of rice and scrambled egg and the vegetables that, after a brief dalliance, she was already learning to refuse. She ate happily. Her eyes were attentive: I could sense, even then, that she understood more than she could express. But she did not sign for more.

In her progress towards walking, Laura was more successful. By the late spring, she was able to flop over and roll everywhere, something we delighted in, if briefly. It was cute, it was progress, but it wasn't a precursor to walking. We wanted her to crawl. Laura *could* crawl, in fact; she just didn't want to. Typical. So I pushed two couches together a Laura's width apart, making a short alleyway. I put her down at one end, on her stomach, and crumpled a sheet of typing paper at the far end, and she crawled towards me. Typing paper was to walking what ranch dressing was to eating: a "motivator," as the therapists call it. Fortunately, the mixed-paper recycling bin was filled with motivators, and I was soon luring my younger daughter with old *New Yorkers*, credit card offers, and the celebrity gossip page of *Parade* magazine. Soon she gave up rolling for the "commando crawl," inching forward on her forearms; then as her arm and trunk strength grew, she crawled on hands and knees, then pushed herself up to a bear walk, and then pulled herself to stand.

By June, Laura could stand, tottering, for a second or two at a time.

She could climb the two steps from the bathroom landing to the kids' room. Her crawling was faster. She could reach more; she *wanted* more. I remembered how Ellie's development had proceeded: not in a simple, steady line, but from plateau to suddenly elevated plateau. By eighteen months, of course, Ellie was much further along. But that comparison seemed increasingly unimportant.

We lived a life of pratfalls, Laura and I. A cartoon life, in the shadow of caricature.

Scene 1: fall from chair, tears, silly Dad, all better.

Scene 2: reach for outlet, Dad swoops down, hollers No no no, lifts her away, no problem, silly Dad, all better.

Scene 3: Dad walking across campus, Laura cradled in left arm. Just goofing around, Dad making faces, Laura laughing. It's the end of the week, late on Friday: Ellie's at gymnastics class on campus, we're meeting Theresa for coffee, and the sun's even come out! Dad gives Laura a big impulsive hug. Then Dad looks up, sees drained face of young woman with backpack, who approaches and asks, hesitantly,—Did you know—do you see—and Dad notices, in that moment, that the diaper has leaked on an epic scale. It extruded its contents, I realize, at the precise moment I was happily squeezing Laura towards me. Home, home, rush home, there's forty minutes before Ellie's gymnastics class ends, enough time to call T on the cell, cancel the half hour of Actual Conversation, get home, strip, bathe, change, return, and on the drive home I am swearing, livid with the stupidity and humiliation of it: the Competent, Affectionate Caregiver, his arm covered in filth. She is the Roadrunner, I am Wile E. Coyote. I am a magnet for anvils. I plummet into canyons.

I long ago established an informal Richter scale for diapers. The critical parameters are quantity, texture, odor, and context. Mild overflow, several hours after a big snack of olives, is a 9. Severe overflow is a 10. Severe overflow at 20,000 feet, with turbulence, and a peeved

United Airlines flight attendant asking you to return to your seat, is an 11. There have been only a few 11s in my years at home with my daughters, and this is one of them.

What I like about cartoons is the ease and convenience of everyday life. It's what I miss, living in the world of love and hindrance. I like the way the characters get dressed, a blur, a fast-forward, and *boom*, they're in tuxedos, they're in drag. I like the precise silhouettes they leave in walls when they're in a hurry. I like the blur denoting work: *zip zip zip*, and Coyote's roadblock is up and ready. That he always loses does not diminish his technical skill: if he had to put in a nose tube, he'd just throw it in the child's general direction, and it'd thread itself right in.

And when things go wrong, Coyote always recovers. Squashed like a pancake, he waddles away, returns at his full height, and when the bundle of dynamite explodes in his hands, he is blackened, tattered, and whole. No violence is great enough to end his life, no humiliation great enough to end his persistence. In real life, Coyote is a bitter old man in an assisted living facility, swearing at *America's Funniest Home Videos*, but in his true element he lives forever, and though flattened, pummeled, burned to a crisp, he springs up middle-aged, hopeful, and good as new. He knows how to endure. Minus the explosives, he'd make a decent at-home dad.

July 2002

It's summer again, Laura's second summer, the sweet weather we endure the rain for. The students go away and give us back our parking spaces. The neighborhood's quiet. Theresa finally gets some time in the lab, a respite from teaching and committee work. A year ago, she received a five-year grant from the National Institutes of Health. It was a bright spot, just before the heart surgery. Now she has to get results. She has to publish, because tenure depends on it. Being Theresa, she doesn't complain about the stress; she works hard so she can get home in time to be with us. But the stress is there.

Laura's not sleeping well, just like Ellie at the same age. We're bleary, but it doesn't matter so much; we don't have school and a dozen activities to get to. The winter viruses are gone too, and the jitters following Laura's April pneumonia have faded.

Ellie sleeps in. When she wakes up she comes downstairs, sits groggily at the bowl of Cheerios I push in front of her. I set Laura in the high chair, dump a can of mandarin oranges on the tray, and say to Ellie, "Miss Smith, take a letter." And in her newly discovered cursive, Ellie writes down the day's list of tasks. I dictate between sips of coffee. I empty the dishwasher, then hoist Laura away from the ruins of her breakfast, brushing off fragments of orange for the dog to eat.

"Oh, Ellie, we need butter. Put down butter."

She writes *buter*. I tell her that *butter* has two *t*'s. She wedges in an extra *t*.

"Oh, Dad," she says. "We need sunscreen."

"Okay," I say, "put that down." I inspect the list and say, "Excellent, excellent, very nice writing." On another day I might say not to write pictures all over the list, but today is a good day.

We change a diaper, Ellie clowning above Laura to keep her from flopping over in midchange. I call the hospital to get the results from Laura's chest X-ray (a follow-up, from her late-spring hospitalization—it's clear), and then we head out on the circuit: Winco Foods, the compounding pharmacy for Laura's heart medicine, the Parks & Rec office to sign Ellie up for T-ball. Then Dairy Queen, because it's a good day. We go on, in and out of car seats, crossing off tasks as we go, and when we come home we fold laundry and Laura falls asleep and takes a long nap and Ellie decides to count to a thousand and ten and I get to write for an hour and a half. When Theresa gets home we report the good things we have done. Everybody is happy, and the kids fall asleep early. It's a lucky life.

A rosy picture. There were days, too, when I woke from nightmares to find resentment sparking like a downed wire. On those days I could see Ellie wondering if my mood was her fault. When I came to myself, I tried to make it right.

I didn't get much done that summer. The bathroom was still unfinished, and writing was slow. We had lost our babysitter, the college student who'd watched the girls off and on since the spring. She was conscientious, sweet, terrific with the girls, and for weeks, without our knowing, she had been telling Ellie the good news about Jesus. We discovered this on a camping trip with two other families, when Ellie sat with her younger friends at a battered state park picnic table, proudly sharing a scrambled story that involved animals on a big boat, talking vegetables, and the son of God who died but didn't die. From the standpoint of experimental psychology, it might have been interesting to see if the confused proselytizing at that picnic table developed into an independent religion. It would have had a six-year-old prophet, two four-year-old acolytes, and an up-and-coming saint with Down syndrome, and by the time Ellie and her friends were done with it, the talking vegetables would probably have been shoved overboard with the animals, to feed the pink sharks. But after the brief *kerfuffle*, as Theresa called it, we moved on.

Having lost the few hours a week of childcare, I slumped back into the usual time-killing strategies: errands, park, more TV than usual. We sat out on the deck, reading in the shade under a tarp. Ellie was in a Berenstain Bears phase, devouring blandly moral tales about visiting the dentist, nightmares, and strangers. The Berenstains were a normal family, except for being bears. They lived in a tree, in Bear Country. The children, Sister Bear and Brother Bear, played with Game Bears and Bearbies. They had a wise, alert Mama Bear who stayed home all day in her polka-dotted housecoat, and an oafish, woodworking Papa Bear, a screwup who meant well. Mama Bear was the core of the family, the dependable one. She hardly ever left the tree.

We did not live in a tree, but our deck was built around one. Theresa had stretched a blue tarp between its lower branches and the low fence surrounding the deck, tying it in place with granny knots. She had set out books, art supplies, bubbles. I had planned something elaborate, a multilevel play structure in redwood or cedar, but Theresa just went out one evening with the tarp and some twine, and it was done.

There is an irritable exhaustion specific to primary caregivers, in the late afternoon, when you are sleep-deprived, caffeine has lost its power to revive you, and you have not had childcare for days. You have already played Chutes and Ladders and Hi-Ho! Cherry-O and Masterpiece, and each time it has taken more time to find and set up the game than it has to actually play it, and somewhere beneath the increasingly snappish exchanges between you and your children, your brain is sinking to the benthic depths of four o'clock, where the last few caffeine molecules, like phosphorescent sea-creatures, are slowly winking out.

Once, when we lived in North Carolina and I was still new at full-time parenting, I tried giving up. Ellie was about a year and a half old then; I was exhausted, and she had refused to nap. So I stuck her in the crib, raised the rail, lay down on the floor, and fell asleep. She yelled and woke me up. I told her to sleep, and she yelled louder. So I took every stuffed animal I could find and filled the crib. Then I lay down and closed my eyes. Ellie threw the animals at my head. They fell with soft thumps around me. When they stopped falling, the crib rail began to rattle. I gathered the animals in armfuls and heaved them back into the crib. In this way I assembled forty-second naps into a simulacrum of rest.

I had quit my job teaching college English. I was retired, at thirty-two.

My dad had died the year before. Even then, it seemed obvious that my quitting work, though he would've hated the idea, was a cockeyed homage to him, an invocation of his practical, data-based spirit. I presented the decision, to myself and others, as if I were arguing the case to him: It was a simple equation. It was economics. We were basically living on Theresa's salary anyway; my part-time teaching job mostly went to paying for daycare. Why not cut the knot? Why not quit, take care of Ellie myself, and write during her naps?

Theresa knew it wasn't that simple. She said: "You may be burned out on teaching now, but you can burn out on taking care of kids too." I said: "I know." She said: "We can afford it, but we might have to dip into savings." I said: "No no, I think we can do it. We'll eat out less."

As practical as my arguments were, what I felt was beyond argument: a wish to reduce life to its essentials. For a year I had watched my father dying in time-lapse. I wanted to build something against that slow catastrophe, to honor family against the loss of family. I must have been convincing. We stood in the almost-finished kitchen, on the new floor, in the yellow light of the new range hood, and Theresa said, "If you're sure," and I felt a flush of renewal to equal the emptiness of my father's loss.

So we began the reversed traditionalism we still live by. We began a new answer to the question: How do you build a life?

We had the long days free. On the good days I knew what that was worth. I did the things Theresa would have liked to do if she weren't working full time. We went to the science museum, looked at poisonous snakes, played with the bright plastic model of the heart. We rode the little train.

Ellie, curious, good-natured, up for anything, shouldered her father's grief without thinking. She was fifteen months old when I decided to resign my teaching job. Each day brought a new word, a new accomplishment. She was walking already. We played hide-and-seek in the yard as she toddled over rutted clay. We looked at birds together, and she said *bird*.

Walking through tall grass to the pond, carrying Ellie in the backpack, I knew I had established a wilderness of decision inside my own life. I was free. I carried a mirror to look back and see if Ellie had fallen asleep yet. When she fell asleep, I could write. Sometimes I'd let her nap in the carrier, letting my writing time bleed away, minute by minute, as I focused binoculars towards the very top of the magnolia, looking for the warbler I'd heard.

Behind the days, I could hear the faint click of an academic calendar ratcheting along without me. The magnolia petals singed and fell, and the warblers came back, migrating north, and then the wood thrushes settled in, and all the while I was not grading papers, not preparing for class, not agonizing over the difference between a B and a B plus. It was a sweet drifting feeling, at sea but not seasick, the city of work blurring into the horizon.

Theresa always said she could tell what kind of day I'd had by the condition of the house. Usually it was trashed: my desk piled up with drafts and books and index cards, the kitchen floor covered in plastic toys, water boiling on the stove for the dinner I'd started too late. The Portacrib was our kitchen island; trapped on the island was Ellie, wailing. She'd have been stretching her arms up for a half hour. Theresa would come in the kitchen door and lift up Ellie, who nestled gratefully there.

Whether women are naturally better nurturers than men is, to me, an uninteresting question. But Theresa, unlike me, has always had an uncanny sense for children. She does not subscribe, as I do, to the Moody Clown school of parenting—one moment jovial fun dad, the next moment severe. She is steady but not distant, and both of our children still settle into that sureness, at the end of the day, with a kind of relief.

And yet it would be too easy to milk the stereotype of Incompetent Dad. I was not Papa Bear. I did fine, and mostly enjoyed it. I had an apron (nonflowered), but then so did my father. He usually got home just at dinnertime and put the apron over his suit so he could eat with us; it was white, with large black letters that read I GOT MY JOB THROUGH THE NEW YORK TIMES. So the tug of Inner Guy, the resistant whine of the masculine, soon faded. I felt, instead, an out-of-the-wayness. A life difficult to explain.

As with Down syndrome, with its multiple names, none accurate or complete—*trisomy 21, special needs, developmentally delayed*—there was no single, descriptive, accepted label for what I was doing. *Stay-at-home dad* came closest in being purely denotative, and yet "staying" hardly begins to describe the work of raising children. *Mr. Mom* and *house-husband* both imply that the role is intrinsically female, and that the man is an afterthought, a pinch-hitter. *Primary caregiver*, in its bland, jargony institutionality, manages to insult everyone: you might as well be feeding rats in a lab. And if a new name arrives—something neutral, generally accepted, like *engineer*—it will be because fathers raising children at home will have become customary, unremarkable. We are not there yet. For now, the multiple labels show a culture thinking about something new.

But the similarities end there. Despite the occasional feature articles in which men whine about playground snubs and a sense of isolation, at-home dads do not suffer the systematic discrimination suffered by the disabled. The fact that men now can and do get to watch kids, in addition to running the world and getting paid more than women for equivalent jobs, is an *expansion* of the male domain: this is one more thing we get to do, and those of us who do get to stay home are lucky to do it.

Taking care of Ellie at home wasn't about grappling with changing cultural notions of manhood. It was about raising a child, and the experiences involved seemed to resonate with the many stay-at-home moms I talked to: the sheer quantities of time involved; the odd *character* of time, the alternation between hectic minutes and trackless hours; the unshakable belief that one could do no higher work than raising a child right, countered by the conviction, after a long day, that I had accomplished nothing.

Behind this routine, grief began to sweeten. The sense that my father, like a piece of metal, had simply been ground to sparks—this faded, and memories from before the cancer began to return. I only missed him. I knew how much he would have loved Ellie, how much he would have *enjoyed* her spirit, her exuberance just behind a scrim of shyness, and wished he could have seen her. It's a feeling renewed by Laura: each new accomplishment evokes his memory, and his loss.

After years of saying that intelligence per se did not matter so much as human decency and kindness, I had found myself crowing over the least IQ-related advancement. I had zero experience with children or developmental curves, but Ellie's cousin Katie had learned the alphabet by eighteen months. So Ellie did too.

We got things done. We left the house with a to-do list and came back with the items crossed off. We drove to the new Food Lion, a few miles from our house; in the store, I'd let Ellie hold the pencil in her fist, smooth the list across the grocery cart handle, and blacken out MILK, BREAD, CHICKEN THIGHS. In empty aisles, we'd get the cart up to speed and I'd jump up and coast. Or I'd push the cart away with Ellie in it and pretend to be looking for her, as she glided away, then catch up to the cart right before it caromed into the cereal. She hiccuped with laughter.

Driving the winding roads home, I saw a landscape in transition. Everywhere new houses were going up: tobacco farmers were retiring, selling off lots to biotech workers and English professors. The houses went up fast; they had sparse new lawns, like hair implants. Beyond them, now and then, you could see an old farmhouse still standing.

We were part of the influx. We couldn't afford the McMansions and didn't want one, but we were still outsiders: that much was clear. Our little farmhouse, with its two-acre plot, was just past the edge of the sprawl. It was a motley neighborhood—two- to ten-acre lots, one neighbor a microscope repairman, another a fireman, another a teacher at the Friends school. Most were Southerners; we were Yankees. People were friendly, but I was beginning to see that we would never entirely belong: that however many cabinets I built, however I landscaped and gardened, being deeply at home in North Carolina required a history and religion we didn't share. Being at home in the South was not something we could renovate our way into.

I finished the kitchen Mike and I had started. I finished my elegy for my father. As I wrote my way through his death, I realized how much I had learned from him about poetry. In the same way he strove to build a power plant in which each BTU and volt was accounted for, in the same way he engineered structures to hold steam and heat under pressure—machines for the translation of energy—so I sought to build closed systems, poems in which metaphors became not disorder or association, but structure. A poem was a power plant made out of words.

And yet, because my assumptions about writing were purely formal, I wound up avoiding any sense of what the writing was *for.* So my poems were limited to the personal, and to quasireligious categories of darkness, light, and mystery. If they were power plants, they were disconnected from the grid, their turbines humming, powering nothing. This was literally true, in that they were unpublished: though I had spent the last nine years telling my writing students to be more conscious of audience, that writing, though solitary, was a public act, I had yet to fully understand this for myself. But this lesson, too, would wait on Laura's arrival.

I don't regret a minute of raising my daughters at home. I've been extraordinarily lucky to do it. But having turned from my father's kind of life, I saw its benefits: that work, at its best, is a blessing, that it lends structure and meaning to the rote arrivals of daylight, translating the viscous hours into tangible accomplishments. A house. A power plant. A completed task. And yet I half knew what was wholly true: that the intangibles, of words, of the durable and unnamable connections between Ellie, Theresa, and me, were the realest things I had. I knew it as I wrote, in the sense of completion the right word afforded, more satisfying than any dovetail.

I had begun, too, to realize the choice underlying the distractions of the rural dream: the choice between making art and making a life. It was one thing to live among handbuilt cabinets, to keep bird lists and conserve heirloom seeds, all the complications of living simply; but as I have learned, if you want to get pages done, you buy the boneless chicken breasts. Or the TV dinner. Or you pick up pizza.

When we moved to Oregon, we bought a house in town.

We signed at Laura throughout the summer. She did not sign back. But we could see a kind of progress. She had two gestures, which seemed meaningful to her, if private. In the first, she splayed her hand, then tapped her high chair tray with her thumb. We took this to mean *hungry* or *more*. She'd also begun using this sign when we read together. It wasn't random; she pointed, invariably, at what most would think of as the picture's subject. If it was a polar bear she pointed to the polar bear. If it was a house, she pointed to the house.

Another gesture seemed simple, universal: she shook her head, in what looked like *no*. By summer's end, this movement was tinted, increasingly, with meaning. When she was full, and I offered a last spoon of applesauce, she'd grit her teeth and say "Grrrr," turning away with eyes squinched and shaking her head. The movement was increasingly definite, a brisk double shake.

We had gestures, but we wanted a sign. More exactly, we wanted what the sign meant: an ability to imitate. If Laura could copy us, then she could learn. Until that point, there wasn't much to do, except persist. Like appetite, language could not be forced; it could only be cultivated.

Her progress towards walking was easier to see. One day late in August, in the park, she stood independently for thirty-eight seconds. She wobbled, she was obviously scared and excited at once, but she did it. Ellie counted the seconds. When Laura fell down, Ellie ran over and hugged her, saying, "Yay, Laura, yay, good job!" Even at age six, Ellie knew it was a big deal for Laura to do something new, though she did not realize how much Laura's progress depended on her.

Eighteen months before, the differences between them had seemed unbridgeable. One child was normal, the other was not. One child had Down syndrome, the other did not. But as Laura grew and learned, the difference that had seemed so obvious, so unquestionable, faded before the parallels. Each new discovery of Laura's reminded me of Ellie, not at the same age but at the *equivalent* age.

The real difference, this time around, was our consciousness of the process. We were aware, as we never had been with Ellie, of stages within stages, markers, milestones. With Ellie, it was simple. Each day she stood a little longer, and there she was: stable, walking. We felt like lucky witnesses, not therapists. With Laura, we counted the seconds. Laura's development was more likely to be divided into named steps, and the steps were more likely to be quantified. Because Laura received services specified in her Individual Family Service Plan, these steps were further classified into gross motor, fine motor, and adaptive categories, and assigned as six-month or one-year goals. Because we saw therapists regularly, we were a bit more aware of the technical complications beneath those goals, like muscle tone, trunk strength, balance. With Ellie, we learned to speak the language of childhood; with Laura, we became linguists, studying its formal grammar. The rules of understanding.

Early that fall, Laura looked up from her high chair and signed *more*. At my near-hysterical praise, she all but shrugged. Of course she could sign *more*. She would've gotten around to it much sooner, but as it was, her schedule was packed.

We remember the first word—a child saying *light* on an airplane, a child signing *more*—but these arrivals deceive. Understanding soaks in, like water darkening a sponge; it osmoses into outward motions, the longed-for, surprising advance. So on the good days, the unmapped neuromuscular depths yield to repetition and love. On the bad days, you feel like a caveman before a supercomputer.

It's easy to forget how long it took for that first sign to take hold. Months. Theresa remembers these things more accurately than I do: her patience, I think, makes her more at home in the long stretches of time that memory and hope require. But as with teaching Laura to eat, we had to lose hope in order to move forward; we had to sign *more*, not hoping for more. By the time Laura began imitating us, this functional hopelessness was beginning to grind itself apart: things just seemed hopeless, period. The motions became automatic, rote, a tic. We hardly noticed ourselves. And then there she was, tapping her fingertips together, asking for more rice.

As with appetite, the switch lay within Laura. It seems, sometimes, that she holds out on us, perversely, in order to remind us she's not a machine to be programmed. Like her father and her father's mother, she's as stubborn as a brick when her mind is made up, and even more stubborn when it's not. Sometimes I think she's as weary as I am of developmental charts, of the incessant, nagging whisper to advance, advance. She keeps her counsel; she takes the next step when it suits her. Until then, her refusals are concise, deliberate, more expressive than any word.

A Complex Sweetness

In the fall, Ellie began first grade at Jefferson School. She loved her teacher, Mr. Kikuta, who was wry, unflappable, businesslike. In our first parent-teacher conference, he said, "I think I could probably just give Ellie my lesson plans and let her teach herself." Ellie began her second year of piano lessons and began playing pieces for two hands, which she had despaired of ever being able to do. She played soccer, though at that age *soccer* means a seething herd of fluorescent-clad children, all attacking a size 3 ball in the exact way minnows attack a worm dropped in the water. Now and then a child picks flowers on the field during the game.

I had not really thought an ordinary life would be possible, this soon. I had projected endless work, health problems, one child's needs gobbling the days. But as Laura's heart surgery receded in memory, and her other therapies settled into a steady effort, we didn't seem that much busier than other families we knew, and much of what kept us busy were things we chose to do.

One day that November, Ellie asked me if people turn to stone when they die. I explained that they didn't. I assumed at first she was thinking of the denouement of the first Harry Potter movie, in which the evil Professor Quirrell turns to stone and crumbles at the touch of Harry's hands, but then I remembered the book about Pompeii we had checked out from the library the month before, with its weeping villagers, spewing lava, and billowing smoke, and realized Ellie had merged this book in her mind with a recent daytrip to Mount St. Helens. We had stood among the blasted rocks, above the gray lake, and looked directly into the crater. We had watched video of the smoke billowing towards us, heard the staticky radio reports from spotter planes, and seen rivers of red LEDs lighting up on a relief map as a deep voice intoned PYROCLASTIC FLOWS. I explained to Ellie that people did not turn to stone when dead, and reminded her that Mount St. Helens was far away.

By twenty-one months, Laura had learned to sit up, to crawl, to stand, to walk, and to eat. She had also learned a few signs (*book, star, cup*). Given the medical delays of her first year, she was positively rocketing ahead. We had seen progress in speech as well, mainly manifested in the long imaginary conversations she carried on, the toy plastic phone cradled against her ear. She paced back and forth, exactly as I did when talking on the cordless. "Da," Laura would say briskly, stomping around like a tiny Russian mobster. "Da. Da." Then a long string of syllables: "Zubbadeedeeday! Dup, dup, dap." Then she'd toss the phone aside.

It was progress. For a long time, she'd only repeated identical syllables—dadada, bababa. But words, as Laura's speech pathologist had pointed out, are composed of diverse syllables, effortlessly combined. We don't think about it; we'd never thought about the fact with Ellie. But with Laura, the fact was highlighted. To help her along, we would repeat her syllables back to her, then add a different syllable. For months, we had conversations like this:

Laura: Ba ba ba ba ba.
Dad: Ba ba ba ba DA!
Laura: Ba ba ba ba ba.

A template of sorts, a rough draft of future conversations, which might go something like this:

Laura: I like the Life Skills class. My friends are all there.
Dad: Life Skills is good, but the regular class is good too!
Laura: I like the Life Skills class.

But of course we had no idea what the future held. Since we knew that Down syndrome tends specifically to compromise speech, we tried not to expect much. We tried to distinguish articulation from communication. We played games, like passing a ball back and forth, with the idea that turn-taking was a prelude to conversation. Now and then, if we were feeling really ambitious, we'd try to have Laura draw pudding or Jell-O up a straw, in order to build muscle tone in the mouth. But we were half burned-out from Laura's first year of therapy, and we weren't convinced the straws were all that important anyway. Laura's muscle tone seemed fine. "Zubbadeedeeday."

She was learning, and that was enough. Her walking was steadier too. She toddled across the living room towards Ellie, who counted steps. By Thanksgiving, fifty-one was the record. It felt efficient somehow, Laura working on gross motor, Ellie working on math.

It's easier to write about development than a child. There are records, for one thing: a child with Down syndrome is nothing if not documented, and so in the reams of progress reports and Individual Family Service Plans and Individual Education Plans, the writer has a handy chronology of milestones. And yet development matters less to me than identity: what a child can do is only part of who she is. That identity, as Laura got older, was increasingly distinct—though, predictably, there was a tension between who Laura was, and who she was supposed to be.

Since Laura's diagnosis, I'd heard from strangers and professionals alike that people with Down syndrome were "sweet." I resisted the idea. It seemed, like the most dangerous falsehoods, just true enough to be believed. Laura *was* sweet most of the time, in her Laura way—impulsive, affectionate, exuberant, giggling and signing *more* at my clowning. Or drowsing against Theresa on the yardsale couch, her left ring and middle fingers in her mouth, her right hand twirling Theresa's hair into knots and curls. Or tagging along after Ellie on the playground, with her newfound wobbling steps. It was a complex sweetness, not the saccharine of diagnosis. It was hers alone.

It's a delicate business, bringing up the problem of stereotype. It positions the writer as prosecutor, the reader as squirming, guilty perp. So let me just say that on the specific charge of thoughtless prejudice in the first degree, I grant whatever immunity is in my power. If you have believed, all these years, that people with Down syndrome are invariably sweet and happy, then fine, no worries, have no fear. Just be open to another point of view, is all I ask. Consider, for example, the other stereotype of people with Down syndrome: that they're stubborn. How can both be possible? If they are stubborn most of the time, or half the time, can they still be counted as sweet? Are they sweetly stubborn, or stubbornly sweet? To claim both is to see that the stereotypes are self-canceling. A group that is both sweet and stubborn sounds almost like an individual, contradictory and complex. Almost.

Laura, we were finding, *was* both—sweet, with an asterisk—and yet, in the details of her behavior, she tended to destroy the stereotype, not fulfill it. "They are not passionate or strongly affectionate," wrote John Langdon Down—a sentiment echoed, in decades since, with words like *docile* and *trainable*—and yet Laura was nothing if not passionate, a child who lived every mood to the fullest. If Ellie needed to practice the piano, Laura would invariably perch on the piano bench next to her, mashing white keys above Ellie's first melodies. Often she was content to play a little while, then be distracted. But sometimes—wanting only to be next to Ellie, to play with Ellie, and, I suspect, not to be *managed*—she'd flail as I lifted her from the piano, then howl when I clicked the baby gate shut.

The mood didn't last. There's a cleanness to Laura's anger: she doesn't smolder, she flares, and when she's done with it, she's done. This has been, over the years, a good lesson to a father who tends to brood, to dwell *on* rather than *in*, to keep the pilot light of anxiety burning. It's a cliché, I know, to talk about how much my kids have taught me. But the cliché is (as my writing students used to say, defensively) true.

Having expressed herself (the gate rattled, the board book thrown, the yell fully voiced) Laura would turn pensive, solitary. She'd sit in the big green armchair, a child potentate, examining a book of signs. I left her alone. I cooked dinner. Around quarter past six, the front door would open, and Theresa would come in, her coat dripping with rain. Each time, Laura looked as if the sun had risen in the doorway.

That December, we flew back East—or was it home? Like most of our friends (information workers, far-flung from the towns that spawned us), we face the seasonal challenge of meeting with two sets of families, and keeping everyone happy. We long ago settled on a standard two-week plan. We fly to Newark, rent a car, then spend about thirty-six hours with my mom in northern New Jersey. Then we go to Pennsylvania for seven to ten days. Then we return for about forty-eight hours with my mom. There are ways to justify this—for example, there are four families to see in Pennsylvania, and one to see in New Jersey—but basically, we do this because it works. The girls play with their cousins; they get to see their Obachama, Aunt Lisa, and Aunt Nina; and if the visit is carefully managed, we leave without regrets.

Since my dad's death, my mom has put up a small Christmas tree each year. It seems out of place somehow, like a bauble fallen in the snow. The townhouse my parents moved to, after I left for college, is spare. The furniture is Scandinavian, not Colonial; the walls are white, as are the miniblinds. The decorations are few, and secular: a faded Cézanne reproduction, my father's engineering license, a wall of diplomas along the stairs.

I didn't grow up there, and I couldn't live there. But when I walk in the door, the place feels like home. Or, more exactly, like a dreamed version of home, the way you fall asleep and wake up in a home that is yours, and not yours. The furniture I grew up with, the teak coffee table and worn velvet chair and tweedy brown couch, seem displaced. It is as if they had never really settled in. As if, since my father's death, they have been poised on tiptoe, waiting to leave themselves.

The first thirty-six hours go okay. No one says anything irreparable. Ellie is polite, a little cautious. My mother seems genuinely happy to see Laura. She asks about our flight, and presses food on us. The refrigerator shelves are sagging with food, with bagels and lox, store-bought sushi, half-gallon cartons of orange juice, a slab of London broil. Soup is on the stove, tiny tofu cubes simmering in broth; the battered pot of rice is on a trivet. I lug our things to my mom's room, which she insists we take; we spread out mattresses on the floor for the girls. I walk upstairs and down, inhaling like a dog. A sharp mothball scent fills the closets, where my father's cardigans and slacks hang empty. My mom sets out dish after dish on the dining room table. We do our best to eat.

We try to help my mother with her computer. She bought it after my father's death, and it runs on a Japanese version of Windows. The effects of this hybridization have been intractable. She can't receive attachments, and her e-mails are filled with slashes, random numerals, character-sized rectangles. She has lugged the computer back to the store, paid too much for unacceptable service. She has buyer's remorse. She thought the Japanese DOS would make things easier. Theresa works on it for a while, but without success.

And then we drive the rented car down to the Philadelphia suburbs to visit Theresa's family. Mike, Theresa's brother, is home from Virginia. Her sisters Bonnie, Susie, and Karen, and their families, all live ten minutes away. Back in Pennsylvania, I can see, Theresa is glad to see them all, a little sad we live so far away. The cousins (at last count, eleven in all) form an instant wolf pack. Its alliances shift, but it is always one pack, and it is always loud. Ellie disappears into sleepovers while we're there. In each house, Laura is wired, radiant, a celebrity. Theresa gets caught up in gossip and reminiscence, and her voice slips sometimes into the accents of her childhood, Pittsburgh vowels and slang, *yins*, the plural for "you." There are elaborate gift rituals, complicated schedules for shuttling children to in-laws. On Christmas Eve, everyone goes to Mass, except for Neil and me, the two nominally Jewish sons-in-law. We sit around in jeans, drinking coffee and talking. All around us is the fluster of children being hurried in and out of bathrooms and into frilly clothes, the last-minute phone calls from whoever is running late and wants someone to reserve a pew, and hurried instructions to Neil and me about what foil tray comes out of the oven when. Then the sudden silence of Jews tending a ham.

This is the family I inherited, with the stories Ellie is beginning to learn, that we expect Laura to learn one day. Though she does not understand everything said to her, she is happily awash in the days, and though she has trouble pronouncing the names, she knows who her cousins are. They love her and accept her for who she is, as children tend to when adults set the right example. Children are quicker to learn this than adults. They do not go through agonizing curves of self-examination; whatever their initial reactions, most, with guidance, move quickly to an uncomplicated acceptance. So it was no more unusual for all of Laura's cousins to accept her than it was for Ellie to do so. It would've been stranger if they hadn't.

We spend a week and return to New Jersey, hoping things will still be okay. But the weather has changed. My mom is trying, she really is, but it is still too soon since Laura's birth. Or the depression since my father's death has not lifted. Or the traumas of growing up in wartime—the unimaginable, which she lived through, and tried to imagine, into a language that stayed too strange to her—have changed her, embittered her, in ways she does not, or cannot, explain.

Or she is just being Mom.

She says, hopefully: "Did you see, did you see how careful she was when she came to that step?"

"Yes," I tell her. "Yes, I saw."

"And she is so *alert!*"

A pause.

"Maybe," she says, "maybe the doctors were wrong. Maybe she doesn't have Down syndrome."

I say: "She took the step carefully because Theresa spent weeks and weeks teaching her how. And she does have Down syndrome. She does."

She says, "Her eyes are so *bright!*"

Pause.

Then, fervently: "There could be a *genius* in there!"

The next morning, still bleary from a 1:30 A.M. argument with my mother that no one heard—a hissed rehearsal of failures, recriminations, and useful facts about Down syndrome—I got up with my family, accepted a silent ride from my mother to the train station, and headed into the city. It was a familiar ritual—the movement from stop to stop, accelerating past split-levels, vacant lots, gas stations, then decelerating at each platform, to the set masks of commuters. For Ellie and Laura, it was brilliant and new. Ellie, already old enough to sense the tension in the air, was glad to be out of the house. Laura was beside herself with the miracle of public transportation. We got off at Hoboken, bought tickets for the ferry, began crossing the Hudson towards the financial district.

I was born in New York City and grew up in its suburbs. Until 1993 my father worked on the ninety-first floor of the South Tower. Still, I felt like a tourist. I am less of a New Yorker than anyone in my family: my sisters both live there, my father grew up in Queens, and my mother arrived there in 1957 and imprinted on it, like a duckling. "She's a New York girl," my dad said once. He doubted she would ever leave the city's orbit. But I had always looked outward, elsewhere. I wanted a story with trees in it.

We had a few minutes before heading uptown to meet friends. As we walked along the cyclone fence, looking into the scoured crater,

Ellie asked me if the men had flown the planes into the buildings on purpose.

I said that they had.

She said, "Well, they should go to jail!"

I said, "Honey, they died."

"Oh," she said.

I told her, "Your grandpa used to work there, but he got transferred in 1993, before the first bombing."

We had been thinking about Down syndrome, not 9/11—or perhaps Down syndrome was a change in life, and 9/11 was a change in climate. In September, fifteen months before, I'd watched the South Tower collapse live, on TV, as Ellie organized her backpack for a first day of kindergarten. In the picture I took that morning, she is smiling widely in front of Jefferson School, and the flag behind her is already at half-mast. A sunny, crisp, early fall Oregon day. Laura was just starting to eat again.

I looked on the memorial plaque for familiar names, and found Fred Kuo, an engineer friend of my dad's. He'd visited the house in the late stages of my dad's cancer, and they'd chatted about the office my dad had left. Something in Fred's manner acknowledged the situation's gravity without making anyone uncomfortable. A rare gift. My father told me, later, that he wanted Fred to have his programmable calculator, and to pick out whatever reference books he wanted.

We left New Jersey the next day. I had a fellowship coming up in February, to spend two weeks at a cabin in the woods, writing the book I'd begun thinking about while Laura was still recovering from surgery. Back home, steelhead were surging upriver. I'd checked the hydrograph on the Internet: there'd been a winter storm, but both the Alsea and the Siletz were dropping back into shape. Cold rivers, the banks dense with ferns and blackberry vines, everything I moved out West for. I thought maybe if the rain held off and Theresa was okay with it, I might get to disappear for an entire day.

Writers and Families

Just before Laura's second birthday, I left for the cabin in the woods. I drove east, like a disoriented pioneer. A few miles beyond Santiam Pass I turned off towards Blue Lake. It had once been a family resort, but a Portland advertising magnate had bought it, renamed it "Caldera," and built A-frames for artists and writers to work in. In the summer, it was a performing arts camp. Walking through the woods one day, I came across an enormous, half-completed outdoor stage.

When I pulled in, a painter was packing up a van with California plates. Otherwise the place was empty. I began unloading the car, dawdling a little. Except for distant diesel rigs growling across the pass, it was quiet. Not the ticking quiet of finishing a paragraph before the sitter left, or the quiet between the skinned knee and the rising howl, but the quiet of the day stretching out before me. There was no soccer practice, toddler group, piano lesson, or cardiology follow-up to get to. There were no DVDs to return. The calendar was empty, as if I had shaken it and the appointments had fallen off.

Each day I woke early, made coffee, then wrote until late morning. Then I quit to go fishing. I drove through sparse Ponderosa forest to the river, where the blue-winged olives were hatching: tiny, drab little mayflies, drifting on the current to dry their wings. They either flew away in time, or got eaten, the trout nosing to the surface and sipping them in. Sometimes I caught fish, sometimes not. Around the time my toes got numb, I drove into town and wrote for the rest of the afternoon.

It had been weeks since my mother and I had spoken, but I had been thinking about her. I had been reading her unfinished memoir.

She had sent it the year before, along with a letter, which begins, "I have written this for you three children who had not had a chance to really know my background." She continues, "This is Part one and I brought it up to the war. For you, probably, the second part would make more sense and meaningful." She also asks for editorial comments, which I did not provide.

A few days into the residency, I called my mother and asked permission to quote from her memoir in my book about Laura.

She sounded surprised, almost desperately happy. She agreed to my request. "Yes, yes," she said. "Of *course*! Use whatever you need!" She asked how my book was going. She was glad I had some time to work. It was difficult, she knew, to write when you had small children.

In an A-frame in Central Oregon, in a house far from home, I sat with my mom's laboriously hand-corrected pages. I read what she wanted her children to know.

The title page read *Remembering How Things Were*. Reading it was less like memoir than time travel. My mother writes, sometimes, as if she were a child again—inquisitive, lonely, mischievous, mystified by the adults around her—and sometimes from the present, on the other side of regret. She remembers her beloved older brother, who died during the war. He looked after her, and drew cartoons for her and her friends; a "cat gentleman" was her favorite. She remembers misfortunes, each one the seed of a present unhappiness: a bad experience swimming, after which she never learns to swim; an early illness, which set her back forever in school.

The memoir is less chronological than spatial. Though she meanders as far back as her earliest childhood memories, and occasionally strays forward into the war, she always returns to her childhood house. Seventy years later, it is as if she were walking through its corridors and rooms. It is a memory palace, where every room has its event: the room where her mother's ashes were, the tall dresser where the doll forbidden to her was kept. She takes time to explain customs of entry, the Japanese names of things: *shoji, geta, genkan*. In describing the house, she gives the measurements of rooms, the height of the front step or a mail slot, the width and depth of the bomb shelter in the yard. The living room was six tatamis wide. She remembers the man who came to repair the tatami mats, the fresh smell of the grass. It is as if she were sketching blueprints for a vanished world.

When she was four, her biological mother died in childbirth, along with the baby. Until he remarried, her father, against the practice of his time and place, became what we would now call a stay-at-home dad. Although she bitterly opposed my own decision to quit teaching and stay at home with Ellie, my mom's few happy memories from early childhood are of being cared for by her father. She recalls a thunderstorm when they sat together in the corridor, and he made up games and stories to distract her from being afraid. She says, in passing, that she likes a corridor in a house.

She remembers that her father liked to fly-fish, that in late May he would disappear, for days sometimes, into the mountains. But after his first wife's death, he sank a *hibachi* in the yard, filled it with water and live fish, and fished in that. Sometimes, while my mother played in the yard, he would fish from inside the house, poking the fly rod through the window.

I called my mother to confirm this, and to ask what kind of *hibachi* could hold fish.

"Not a *hibachi* like Americans use for cookouts," my mother told me. "More like a big porcelain bowl. Maybe two or three feet wide, and pretty deep."

"What kind of fish did he put in it?" I asked. "Goldfish?"

"Yes, goldfish," she said. "Also *fana*."

"What's *fana*?"

"Ahh . . . " she says, the way she does when she's riffling through a mental phrasebook. "Snapper," she says finally.

I don't know what this fish looks like. I've been fishing since I was eight—an obsession, like baseball, that mystified both of my parents—and I know striped bass, bluefish, flounder, largemouth bass, small-mouth bass, bluegill, pumpkinseed, crappie, bullhead, rainbow trout, brook trout, brown trout, cutthroat trout, bull trout, and mountain whitefish. The juvenile bluefish I used to catch in tidal estuaries were called *snapper*, and so are the red, glaucous-eyed corpses at the fish counter, marooned on stained ice chips under curved glass. I am unable to imagine either one circling inside a porcelain container buried in a yard in a Tokyo suburb in prewar Japan.

In the mountains, my grandfather fished for *ayu*, which my mother describes as "silver." She remembers the creel her father brought them home in. Later, she said, he bought a special Thermos. A Thermos full of *ayu*. I couldn't picture it. (Later, I Googled "ayu." It looks like a cross between a trout and a sardine.)

She left Japan in 1957. She had intended to get a college degree, attend graduate school, and get a job here, perhaps as a teacher. She had not meant, she told me once, to become a housewife. While getting her bachelor's degree in English at Columbia, she had met my father, who was getting a master's degree in mechanical engineering, but was expanding his horizons in an art appreciation course. The family legend has it that she helped him write papers for art class, and that he helped her pass astronomy. They married in 1963. I was born in 1964, my twin sisters in 1967. Afterwards, she said, my father wanted her to be at home. When my sisters and I were young, she began taking fiction workshops at Columbia with William Owen, a memoirist and folklorist. What began as a short story soon became a novel. Owen encouraged her to publish.

The novel is called "The Sun Was Going Down," and its subject is a squadron of kamikaze pilots during World War II. By the time I was in middle school, it had gone through two drafts, and was five hundred pages long. I have not read it. When I was a boy, I was told that the book "contained adult material," and as I got older, I turned to poetry. So her book became, like so much else about my mother, both deeply familiar and completely unknown. In this it was like Japanese itself, which was everywhere in the house—on bags of rice crackers and containers of tea and the crinkly blue airmails that came from Japan, and, infrequently, in my mother's voice, when she spoke to someone overseas. I was always amazed at the transformation: speaking Japanese, she seemed twenty years younger. She was happy, animated, fluent, at home.

In the late afternoons she would turn off the typewriter and start dinner. From the TV room, my sisters and I could hear the colander banging in the sink, a wooden spoon rapped sharply against a frying pan. She would call us in to set the table, and we wouldn't answer. We were watching *Star Trek*, which began at 6:00. Dinner was at 6:30, when my dad got home. *Star Trek* was over at 7:00. We had seen every show three times over, but we still dragged our feet. We were, in her words, ungrateful and lazy. During the war, she had eaten grass. During the war, her mother's wedding dress had been sold to a farmer for a sack of rice. These things fascinated me, but not in the context of being nagged, particularly when Captain Kirk had not yet finished off the Gorn.

Since the book was never published, it is easy to say, in retrospect, that the decision to write it was unwise. Why not, in the best workshop tradition, *write what you know?* Why write about an insular, suicidal culture she could know almost nothing of? Why, for that matter, write in English? Why compete with a country full of writers? It seems a classic instance of overreaching. And yet writing her novel may not have been a momentous decision, so much as a choice that deepened. She may only have waded in until the shore was far from sight.

There is nothing lonelier than an experience unshared: the secret, held behind the force fields of memory and language and culture. To write a novel about that time was, perhaps, a way of breaking down invisible barriers. Not only the ones between herself and her uncomprehending neighbors, or between herself and her American children, but between herself and a world *she* could not have known: the world of men at war, a world she could only imagine, as she sewed buttons onto officers' uniforms and counted out pills into bottles. The world of her older brother.

She shut the study door and wrote. She turned away from her family and reached out to an imagined public. Which is what I was doing, miles from my family, at once missing them and relishing the quiet hours. Like my mother before me, I was trying to carve out time, a meaningful existence in work; like her I faced the world by turning away, choosing contact and distance at once. In this, writing is like raising a disabled child: one is always a little bit removed, and a little bit on stage.

Years ago, I called my mother and asked if I could read the novel. There was a long silence on the phone; it was as if she had not heard me. I asked again; another silence. Then she changed the subject.

I was absolved. I did not ask again. A few weeks later, she brought it up. She apologized, saying she had been so surprised, she hadn't known what to say. But she didn't want me to read it yet; she still had some changes to make.

I wrote in the rhythm of burning pine, the blue-winged olive hatch, of caffeine cresting and fading in the blood. Each morning I woke to a cold house, stood on the freezing slates by the woodstove, and lit the fire. I turned on the little radio—the northeast corner of the cabin got the best reception—then made coffee and began to write. In the late morning I'd shut off the radio, then drive down washboarded forest roads to the river.

One day, fishing nymphs, I hooked a fish that took almost all of my line out. He got broadside to the current and shot downstream. Then the line went slack. When I reeled in, there was a single hexagonal scale on the point of the hook. A whitefish, swiping at the fly, then turning away too late. I sloshed out of the river towards the Subaru, peeled off the waders, broke down the rod, drove into town with the heater on full. I sat in Angeline's, sipping coffee, writing about chromosomes, about my mother's memoir, about the Christmas visit gone wrong.

I wondered whether we would be estranged permanently. It seemed at least possible: Laura's arrival had catalyzed a reaction difficult to reverse. It seemed sometimes what was left between us was pulled tight and thin as DNA itself—a narrow cable, stretched across the continent—and Laura's arrival had stretched that cable to its tensile limits. At what point, I wondered, do the bonds break? What word, like an enzyme in a test tube, is powerful enough to scissor the strand in two?

As I thought about our story and how to tell it, I worried less over sentences than questions of right and wrong. I'd written poems about family before; I'd written about my Japanese grandfather, and about my mother's life as a writer; I'd even set these stories against the unending story told by DNA. But I could no longer take refuge in art and implication. I wanted to make things plain, and as a result, there were ethical implications impossible to ignore. I wondered if, by telling the story, I could make that story a tragedy. I wondered if, with my meditations on inheritance, I might wind up disowned. All seemed possible.

I wrote in Angeline's until closing time. A Northwest version of the solitary work I grew up with: my father in the attic, studying an intricate map of pipes and ducts; my mother in the study behind closed glass doors, typing her novel. A state of mind balanced between loneliness and solitude. I missed Theresa and the girls, most of the time.

It is easy to decide to write a book, as easy as deciding to renovate a house. But in writing, as in renovation, there is the sobering moment when the project's true dimensions become visible.

After years of writing poetry—reading the grain of a word, dovetailing it to another—prose had been, at first, a relief. If poetry was cabinetmaking, prose was frame carpentry. There were structures, plans, things to look up. There were *tools*: Hi-Liters in all colors, paper clips large and small, index tabs, accordion files, scissors, glue sticks, Scotch tape, hole punchers, binder. Two years into my book, I finally had everything on Ellie's kindergarten supply list. I scissored printouts to pieces. I color-coded the pieces, and glue-stuck them to sheets of paper, and hole-punched the paper, and put it in the binder. I scribbled prospective schema in a pocket notebook, on scrap paper, and once in sidewalk chalk, as the girls and I played outside. I forgot to transcribe it, though, and that night it rained.

We Estreichs—particularly my mother and I—have a way of getting in over our heads. We are perfectionists *and* digressionists, the worst combination possible, and we take on projects whose completion recedes, miragelike, towards the next crest in the road. It may be that difficulty is the point. "Life is pain," my mother told me once, "so you might as well work." The words distilled her. I put them in a poem, in the book that took me years to write.

She did complete the novel. She had an agent; according to her, the book was almost published. I wonder, sometimes, how things might have been. After the last rejection, she stopped writing for a long time. She worked in the city, in a Japanese bank in the North Tower. We used to joke that she and my dad could wave to each other. She had to bring tea to executives. It was the precise sort of subservience she had tried to leave behind in Japan: she once told me she hated the way everyone said *sumimasen*, "excuse me," as if apologizing for their very existence. *Sumimasen, sumimasen*, she said, mimicking a cringing etiquette. She disliked the bank, and came home muttering "JJMCP, JJMCP," which stood for Japanese Jingoistic Male Chauvinist Pig.

All the same, my mother had wanted me to do something profitable and respectable: banker, ambassador, lawyer. We argued often about it, while I was in college and after. All along I consoled myself that she knew these were ludicrous suggestions for me, that she was secretly pleased with my choice to write. But at Caldera, with one unpublished manuscript, and a half-finished one expanding in all directions, I began to entertain a more disturbing possibility: that she had actually known what she was talking about. That she wanted to protect me from her unhappiness, knowing how easily a small ambition can expand to a large one, and a large one decompose into bitterness.

On the coffee table, beside an optimistically large pile of reference books and Xeroxed articles, sat a college textbook entitled *Introduction to Genetic Analysis*. I had dragged the textbook along—pursuing my teeny, personal grail of genetic literacy, a shadow of the Grail in every cell—but every time I tried to read it, I glazed over. It was clear I did not have the expertise, the time, or, frankly, the interest to sustain any meaningful level of study. I was trying to write about my daughter, to tell her story and our family's story, and the specifics of ribosomes or mRNA or tRNA did not really matter that much. Laura had been with us for two years. Whatever the mechanisms were, she would still upend her cereal bowl now and then, just to wake me up.

I had at first turned to the textbook as a source of fact, but it had become more interesting as a source of error. Its description of Down syndrome, even by contemporary standards, was deeply flawed:

> The multiple phenotypes that make up Down syndrome include mental retardation, with an IQ in the 20 to 50 range; broad, flat face; eyes with an epicanthic fold; short stature; short hands with a crease across the middle; and a large, wrinkled tongue. . . . Mean life expectancy is about 17 years, and only 8 percent survive past age 40.

I then had the sixth edition of the textbook, which was published in 1996. The eighth edition (2006) reproduces the description unchanged. In either case, the description is profoundly out of date. IQ is, at best, a partial measure of the abilities of people with Down syndrome. But the estimate in *Introduction to Genetic Analysis* is low to the point of falsehood. Most sources assert that the majority of people with Down syndrome test in the mild to moderate range of retardation—from 40 to 70—and that a significant percentage are in the low normal range. 50 is not the upper limit; it is the mean. Life expectancy, at the time of the sixth edition of the textbook, was not seventeen; it was rapidly approaching fifty.

Beside the text was a line drawing that looked like no human being I knew, but which seemed an exact rendering of what we feared when Laura was born. It was nameless, of course. Its eyes were enlarged, almond-shaped, dark in outline, tilted—half Mongol, half Area 51—and its organs, the defective ones anyway, were visible through its skin. Each was labeled, with a caption in the margin: *congenital heart disease* pointed, with a thin black line, to a heart like a carious tooth; *enlarged colon*, to a fragment of wrinkled tube. *Big, wrinkled tongue* was thrown in for good measure.

Next to the line drawing was an unflattering photograph taken at the Special Olympics. A young woman with Down syndrome is lunging forward with a baton; behind her, slightly out of focus, are two young men, also with Down syndrome. The picture is clearly intended as a sensitive gesture, a reminder of capability and potential. And yet what do these people have to do with the mutant in the line drawing? How, for that matter, should we see them, in light of the text? Do they not have the heart defects, the enlarged colons? They seem to be late in adolescence: are they near the end of their allotted fraction of a score? Or are they, unlike the creature in the line drawing, outliers, anomalous anomalies, healthy overachievers? Which picture should we believe?

In that pair of images, I saw the dilemma of Laura's early days, when I was stuck between two visions of what she might be. In one, she was the Visible Child: her skin transparent, to reveal the defective systems within. In another, she was a child who might have friends and run with a baton.

It was beginning to occur to me that I was on the wrong track. I had been working on long explanations about what Down syndrome *was*, something that—after two years—ought to have been simple enough to write. And yet I could not quite get the explanations right, and I could not make them fit with the story I was trying to tell. Perhaps, then, what Down syndrome "was" mattered less than the way it was described. That chromosomes were real, that science could illuminate their workings, that medicine could apply these lessons, I did not doubt: if not for science and medicine, I knew, Laura would not be alive. And yet when the biological fact was translated into words, something happened. The definition had a shape, a form.

If this was true, then what I knew—as a writer, and a former teacher—was already relevant and useful. I could think of myself not as a poet trying to scale the mountain of science, but as a writer thinking about writing. And then it came to me: I *had* been looking at writing all along. A description is not a syndrome. A description is made of words. The words fell into patterns. I could, I realized, think about the patterns; and I could set those false patterns against the truth of an individual life.

In the evenings I walked to the Data Shack, a slightly-larger-than-outhouse-sized outbuilding with a phone and a 14.4 modem, and dialed my home number. Sometimes I could hear the Little People Playset in the background. My mom had sent it to Laura just before I left for Caldera. It had a house, a motorized circular driveway, a little car, and stubby cylindrical people that fit into the car's matching holes. The boy and girl were named Freddy and Sonya. They had catchphrases. Freddy was blond and had blue plastic overalls molded onto his body. Sonya had dark hair, and seemed intended as Asian. There was a fluty quality to her voice, something in the *r*'s and *l*'s. You could imagine Freddy getting in trouble, but not Sonya. Laura put the girl in the car, in the house. The driveway turned. The house sang a song, which had begun to grate: the toy had no volume control. But as Theresa pointed out, Laura liked it.

But then, Laura had always liked my mom. During the Christmas visit, she often chose her first. Uninterested in the ferocious etiquette of history that Ellie, at six, was uneasily beginning to grasp, she toddled happily past Theresa to my mom. She recognized a familiar when she saw one. My mom, for her part, was clearly happy to have someone go to her without question.

One day, in fourth grade, I announced to a small group of children that my mother was Japanese, my father Jewish. Dawn of a writer: These are interesting facts about me! Others will find them interesting too! There was a day's silence, as if the school were thinking about me. Afterwards, I'd hear, from time to time, "chink" and "kike" called up the street. It was as if an asterisk floated above my head, and "chink" and "kike" were the footnotes.

A small taste, a sip, of an ultimate loneliness. I didn't have words for it, but I felt as if I had been erased from the earth. I knew, without knowing why, or how to say that I knew, that the label provided a profound satisfaction for the labeler. A mystery had been solved; something had been put in its place.

By the time I was nineteen, I did not look so Japanese. I went to Japan to meet my uncles and grandmother. In the weeks before I left, my mother taught me the basic grammars and vocabularies she had tried to teach me as a child. We sat at the dining room table, with the *hiragana* and *katakana* she had written out in black marker. I mispronounced words deliberately and by accident, I made bad jokes, and she stifled giggles like a schoolgirl. I traveled across the ocean, with my rudiments of grammar and my hundred or so words. I met my relatives. In Hakone, on a tram far from the usual tourist paths, children snickered and said *Gaijin*, foreigner. Everywhere, feeling suddenly white and tall, I told people *Hahawa nihondesu:* "My mother is Japanese." Invariably the response was excited surprise, a stream of Japanese words, and then—after I had made my incomprehension clear—the sentiment expressed, in halting English, that it was a shame I had not learned my mother's language.

Each evening I called Theresa from Caldera, but our conversations were hurried. Laura was fussy, Ellie needed help with her homework, it was time for bed. The stress in Theresa's voice told me that my disappearance had its costs.

I have given to my children what my mother gave to me: a loving parent who is preoccupied with a distant goal. For years, Ellie has been able to read the switch from one to the other: I hold up a finger to wait until the paragraph is over, and she obeys. Laura is less patient, more likely to seize the pencil and index card, then run. In the war for attention, she is a brilliant tactician.

A few days before I returned from my writing retreat, I got a letter from Ellie:

> *Dear Daddy I hope you are having a fun time fishing and writeing at Caldera. I hope we can visit you next week. Grandma says that you took more than two pownds of coffee. I usume you did. Laura Is doing pretty well, But she threw up on Sunday night and started gagging. Were all fine Grandma says we* ~~have none noone~~ *don't have anyone to be silly or funny anymore so I'll have to be silly. have you gone fishing yet? I gess you have. I can keep sending you letters If you want. I hope you can see Grandma before she leaves.*
>
> > *yors Sinciry*
> > *Ellie lucille Estreich*
> > *Look on back*

On the back was the elaborate bird-in-a-palm tree all the first graders were learning to draw. Ellie had written above it, with an arrow, "for Daddy"; beside it, with another arrow, "a bird, or a parrot." Just below the bird was a flag, and a caption:

and happy Presidents Day

The Labyrinth of Normal

That April, we drove to the county office to meet with Pat Hill; it was time to develop a new year's Individual Family Service Plan. It was the third of these we'd done, and it had come to seem a sort of bureaucratic birthday, a government-form counterpart to that year's candles and cake. Though, for the first IFSP at least, we had not been in a particularly celebratory mood.

We sat in the toddler classroom on tiny chairs. Laura went immediately to the sand table. She filled a measuring cup, then poured it over a beach toy, making a plastic wheel spin. I remembered Ellie, in our North Carolina side yard, filling metal bowls with a garden hose. The water swirled and glittered and spilled over, and when the bowls were full, Ellie emptied them again. Laura had that look now, a child absorbed in sifting and pouring the tangible world. There was nothing to construct or complete.

We began signing the forms. We confirmed our current mailing address, acknowledged the offering of our rights and responsibilities. Then we began the odd project of dividing our second daughter into developmental categories: fine motor, gross motor, cognitive, adaptive, speech. We read reports and recommendations from Laura's therapists. We decided number of minutes of direct consultation per week and per year; we decided where services would take place. We talked about the Parent-Tot class.

Late in the meeting, in a just-as-a-matter-of-curiosity way, Pat asked us how many signs Laura had. We added them up. *Book, thank you, please, Mom, Dad, Ellie, elephant, French fries, flower, car, bicycle, alli-*

gator, rice, noodles, bread, crackers, eat, drink, dog, cat, bear, monkey, shoes, bath, stars, moon, sleep . . . A board book cosmology, an Eden with carbs. I jotted them down in my shirt pocket notebook, the one filled with cartoon animals, grocery lists, and fragmentary schema for the still-untitled book. Laura had forty-one signs in all.

We had noticed, without really noticing. We had begun to lose ourselves in an ordinary, developing childhood—one where you look back, now and then, startled by how far you've come. Though there was still an aftertaste of *if* in every *when*, a whisper of relief in each new achievement, we no longer really doubted that Laura would learn. It occurred to me that we had been developing too: taking baby steps, learning the rudiments of a language, trying to meet our own adaptive and cognitive goals.

Pat was as pleased as we were, but told us, apologetically, that the forty-one signs would not be recorded in the IFSP. Laura's goals were in speech, so her progress was as unofficial as it was real.

We long ago got used to the bureaucracy. That it exists at all is an achievement of the parents, activists, and occasional enlightened politician of a generation ago. We do not take it lightly, and are grateful that most of the people we've worked with have been, like Pat, affectionate towards Laura, thoughtful, good at what they do. But every celebration is shadowed by comparison. From one point of view, forty-one signs were an enormous achievement; from another, they were simply less than speech. Even in the best of circumstances, it is a dizzying and emotionally draining experience to keep both perspectives in mind; and so I am not surprised when I glance at Theresa and see her knuckles whitening around her pencil.

Once I saw tears interrupt her focus. This was years later, at a meeting with a psychologist for the school district. The psychologist had done an IQ test on Laura, and was going over the results, which would help determine Laura's kindergarten placement. He was a decent man, he liked Laura, he was sensitive to the tensions of the situation, but most of what he had to say added up to deficit: the things Laura could not say, the tasks she could not do, the questions she did not seem to understand. He noticed Theresa welling up and seemed startled, a little unsure of himself.

We live in the labyrinth of Normal. If we could only climb the walls high enough, we could see the maze whole, for the pointless thing it is. But we cannot. In meetings like these, my mind wanders down corridors both dimly lit and familiar. I think about the absurdity of assenting, again and again, to every abnormality, to the obvious fact that Laura is different, so that we can get services to help her develop more, well, *normally*. We are old hands at negotiating the maze now, at retracing the old steps from Present Level of Performance to Placement Recommendations. We do not *feel* lost, and the occasional bureaucratic Minotaur is more obtuse than fierce. But it is hard not to dream of a life without walls, a world where Laura's differences are unremarkable. Where we are free of the obligatory stigmata of IQ tests, assessments, measurements of function: every standard deviation that sets her aside, so she might be included again.

In the meeting, I protested weakly: wasn't Sign a language, just as much as English? But that was not really the issue. Speech was our goal too.

It was a good spring. We stayed out of the hospital; the last of Laura's heart medications, captopril, was finally discontinued; kindergarten was far off. Everything we did was educational. If we played in the park, that was balance and strength, gross motor. If she plucked mandarin oranges from her high chair tray between finger and thumb, that was pincer grasp, a fine motor thing—not to mention the still-live miracle of eating—and if she signed to us, that was language. It was like and unlike teaching Ellie. We turned, more often, in back eddies of development, stalled for a while as the river went past us. But eventually we broke free, rejoined the main current.

We walked to the park, the supermarket, the university, the library. I remembered the days after she was born, when her diagnosis was still half a secret. We were dazed in a dry spring. In the stroller was an infant as light as a chromosome. Now Laura wanted to walk; I brought the stroller for when she got tired. Some days were chilly and damp, but they were moving off. The crocuses had flowered already. The apple trees by the high school filled in, two days of gorgeous pink blossoms, and then a big windy rainstorm tore the petals away. They clogged the sidewalk cracks, lined the curbs, flecked the uncut hair of the park.

It's not the winter-long rain that's hard. I'm used to it now, and though I miss the *precision* of East Coast seasons—green summer, red autumn, white snow—the rain is at least familiar. It is the weather of Holland. Some days I almost like it. I can convince myself of this until maybe March, when the rain starts to fade. Then, in April, we get a whole week of sun, and I am flooded with gratitude and false hope, and then the rain returns. *That* is the most depressing time of all.

We lived a few blocks from the university, in the mix of run-down student rentals, new families, homeschoolers, the retired and widowed. A Pentecostal church sat on the corner and thumped with worship twice a Sunday, and most days you could hear power tools, a landlord fixing up a rental, a homeowner trimming out a window, my neighbor building a cedar trellis to sell. I liked walking around and looking at the yards, a precise index of the neighborhood's mixed demographic: some were grassless, native-plant-filled, ecologically correct; some were scattered with upended toys, Big Wheels and Sit'n Spins and fallen bicycles; some were outposts of order, edged, weeded, and chemically green; and some were overgrown, scattered with beer cans, broken glass, and the odd sofa, its damp stuffing and springs exposed.

It was unlike the suburban towns I'd grown up in, where trains vacuumed commuters from quiet streets in the morning, then disgorged them again in the evening. But I was approaching forty. It's the age I associate with my dad, though he lived until sixty-five. So in me, too, as if a switch had been flipped, I began to think we might not stay. The neighborhood had been changing. It was a little louder on the weekends. Walking Penny, I'd see knots and pods of students, their faces sidelit by cell phones.

We had—not a community, exactly, but a frayed network within a community, one network among many, the seniors, the students, the young families like us. In our four-block-square area, we knew, on average, the residents of one house out of five. I liked going out, seeing people we knew. I'd be out walking with Laura, and we'd run into friends, and sooner or later we'd decide dinner was too much trouble to fix, and we'd be ordering pizza and eating in the park. Events had a way of gathering steam.

Late that spring, I decided to get my hair cut. It had been halfway down my back in high school, had receded to shoulder-length by college, and since then had raised and lowered, like a tide, around my ears. It was getting in my eyes, and I was tired of it. So I walked with a six-pack of Henry Weinhard to my friend Andre's house, two blocks away. On the way, we told people about my plan. "I'm going to buzz it," I said, "just get rid of it all." By the time I was sitting on a kitchen chair in Andre's backyard, we had a small crowd. They kept their distance, as if they might accidentally get haircuts too. Andre plugged in his clippers and clear-cut everything right down to the scalp. I felt like a dog about to have an operation.

When the haircut was done everyone clapped. Then they came forward, to run their palms over the stubble. Theresa had the old look of affectionate resignation. Ellie was pink-cheeked with sympathetic embarrassment. Laura took one look at me, made a long, angry "ahn" of disapproval, and shoved the flat of her hand towards me as if defying an oncoming vampire. Then she said, firmly, "Mum mum," and buried her head in Theresa's shirt.

— ◆ —

I'd come home from Caldera recharged, ready to write, even convinced I would complete the book soon. I was wrong about that last part, as writers often are. But I had also sharpened my focus. I was no longer interested in genetics per se; I was interested in patterns of description, in the way the chromosome's story is told.

When Laura was first diagnosed, I thought there was a single thing called Down syndrome, and that I could find out what it was. I assumed that once I possessed this information, its relation to Laura would be clear. Nothing about Laura undid this assumption: she was a blank screen, on which every fear or fact could be projected. But even in the depths of the ICU, Laura's personality was beginning to appear, and the more she came into focus, the less relevant the projections became. Two years later, the general descriptions and the particular child seemed utterly distinct. If I read about Down syndrome, it was only to understand the fictions by which we live.

I went back to the library. I looked for Down syndrome everywhere. I wandered through the nonfiction stacks, flipping through indexes, where the condition inhabited different alphabetical neighborhoods: in parent guidebooks, it was "development," "diagnosis," "duodenal atresia"; in alternative medicine guides, "Dossey, Larry" and "doula"; in genetics textbooks and books about the Human Genome Project, "DNA," "double helix," "Drosophila Melanogaster." Each new description seemed slightly, dizzyingly different from the others. The thing that once seemed as simple and clear and unitary as a lens had broken into something endlessly faceted, like a compound eye. There was no single, universally accepted definition of Down syndrome; there were only endless versions. And yet from one source to the next, the descriptions had a common pattern. That pattern was the list.

It is the primary way of describing Down syndrome, the way the extra chromosome is expressed. At first, it seems such an obvious and natural choice as to hardly deserve comment. Biology is multiple, and language is linear. The syndrome has hundreds of possible features. What can you do, but state them in order?

But which features should be selected, and how should they be described?

And why is Down syndrome being described in the first place?

Because the answers vary, the lists vary too. Each version tends to be influenced, subtly or not, by the writer's agenda and assumptions. The first list belongs to John Langdon Down, and behind its scrim of objective-seeming observation, his racial preoccupations are easy to see: he focuses on hair ("not black, as in the real Mongol"), the eyes ("obliquely placed . . . The palpebral fissure is very narrow"), and skin tone, which he claimed had "a slight dirty-yellowish tinge." In the same way, today's lists, though apparently objective, tend to be tailored to specific ends. Genetics textbooks class the syndrome with other aneuploidies (variations in chromosome number), while emphasizing phenotypes and mechanisms of nondisjunction or translocation. New-parent guides emphasize possibility and available therapies. Pregnancy guides, depending on their orientation, may emphasize caution, lovability, or horror.

Though things have gotten better over the years, I was struck by the insistently negative tone of many accounts. Slanted language pervades: "chances" become "risks," "characteristics" become "abnormalities," and "mild" or "moderate" become "severe." In many cases, the condition itself is described as a "malformation," an "abnormality," an "error," a "defect." People do not simply have it: they are "victims," they "suffer." Life expectancy is underestimated. Medical problems are exaggerated in severity and frequency. The idea of tragedy, whether through financial ruin or the misery of siblings, is common. Stereotypes of character are presented as biological fact: "sweet" and "happy" are mixed with heart defects and shortened lifespans, as if all sprang equally from the chromosome. Even the word "Mongol," and all its variants, crops up occasionally, as does the odd reference to primates, a vestige of the ugliest strains of twentieth-century eugenics. There are positive notes, but these tend to ring false: "Children are generally trainable," claims *The Signet Mosby Medical Encyclopedia* (1996), "and in many instances can be reared at home."

Reading these descriptions, I felt as if I were back in my old job, teaching freshman comp. The assignment: *Describe Down syndrome in a page or less. The form of the description is up to you, but the information presented should be accurate and up-to-date, and the language you choose should be precise, with attention given to tone and implication. Extra credit will be given to those who remember that conditions inhere in human beings.*

In general, the more recent the list, the more accurate and neutral it tends to be. The best make the developing individual central, not a footnote. But even when these criteria are satisfied, even when the depressingly usual exaggerations are set aside, there are deeper limitations inherent in the form.

Every diagnostic list, by definition, sets the child with Down syndrome apart. Some writers compensate for this divide, and some do not. But in the end, a parent dreams of a time when the divide does not exist in the first place; when we do not need to say *a child first*; when every child is seen as inhabiting a continuum of human abilities; when the idea of "normal" is used in a strict, statistical sense, and not as a divisive, emotionally loaded label; and when that label is invoked only to help the person it describes. These are, typically, insights that parents of disabled children arrive at, simply in order to stay sane. But they are not yet generally accepted.

To be a parent is to keep a story, to nurture another's identity through time. Because of this, a list is at best insufficient to the experience, at worst inimical. A list has no room for story: It is a world without individuals, a world without verbs. There is nothing about what its diagnostic subjects *do*; there is only what they *are*. What they "are," of course, is not up to them. They do not describe themselves; they are only described.

For Laura, speech was slow, but signs were easy. We did what worked. We kept at speech, but we lived by signs.

Every sign filled me with gladness and hope: for the parent of a child with Down syndrome, the future is never far from mind. And yet on any given Tuesday morning, I wasn't thinking about kindergarten, or an independent life. I was having a good time, hanging out with Laura, reading, playing, and—as far as we could—conversing. Whatever her signs signified about the future, they were a definite brightness in the present. I liked the *way* Laura signed; her words, however limited, were *hers*, in a way no IFSP could contain. What moved me was the way she held a word in her hands.

Her signs were a dialect for a country of one. In *alligator*, for example, the signer's arms are jaws: elbows together, the right hand snapping downwards to meet the left. Her alligator lay on its side, its jaws meeting in a single, exaggerated clap. *Phone*, in our house at least, was the mock-Hollywood gesture for *call me*, thumb to ear, pinky to mouth. Laura tilted her head, pressed her fist to her cheek. And in the official sign for *book*, the hands hinge open—the pinkies the book's spine, the palms the text, like a minister holding a Bible. Laura's palms met at the heel, then opened outward, its pages facing the listener. Who knows why? Perhaps she was imagining her own books, whose pages tended to be wider than they were tall. Perhaps, because books were read *to* her, she was pretending to read them to others. Perhaps she simply found her altered signs more comfortable. But once she made a sign her own, she rarely went back.

We didn't correct her. We knew what she meant. We'd begun sign-ing for the usual reasons: a head start on speech, a way for Laura to express herself in the meantime. But that spring, it occurred to me the real benefit of Sign was that it put us, and Laura, on an equal footing: we knew exactly as many signs as she did. It was a visa to her country, a way to visit for a while.

There were pleasures to Sign. To say it enriched life, as if life were only a white bread with vitamins stuffed back in, is not quite right: it was more like an unnamable flavor. A trace, a hint of a process. I liked using *only* Sign. I'd hold up the letter *F*, and bounce it on the air— *French fry*—and her eyes would widen, she'd smile, run to the door and wait, signing, insistently, *French fry! French fry!* It was as if we shared decoder rings.

In time, she began to teach us. She invented signs as she needed them. The first of these, depressingly enough, was *TV*: she'd run to the couch, place the heel of her hand beneath her chin, flick the fingers up. An inscrutable insult; a variation on *pig*. For *library*, she wiggled her in-dex fingers above her head, like rabbit ears; we never knew why. There were gestures, habits, less easily identifiable as signs, but clear nonethe-less. Patting the floor beside her meant *sit down and play with me*. If I was clowning, balancing alphabet blocks on my head then shaking them off, she'd run to Theresa, tug her pant leg, point: *look what he's doing this time*.

So much of our parenting takes place not in the clear light of ar-gument, but in the shadowy territory in and around and between words. Every family has its secret language of gesture and glance and context: the set face that precedes the argument, the exchanged glance that sparks sudden laughter. Laura's presence thrust that language into the foreground. Her signs gave form to the unspoken. But then there was something about her that made invisible things apparent, and lift-ed what was submerged into the light.

— ◆ —

We lived in our Pacific Northwest bubble, our Biosphere with Bike Lanes, with its bronze salmon and drunken college students and still-thriving downtown, with its seasonal farmers' market and bipolar weather and a newspaper where the same six or so cranks wrote in weekly to rehearse their favorite complaints. On a good day, the place has a *Northern Exposure* kind of feel: it is easy to believe, if you don't look hard, that the problems are mild and the people are only quirky. We belong here, more than we have anywhere else, but to have a child with Down syndrome somehow defines a distance between us and our adopted land.

Once, at the opening of the new branch of the food co-op, my friend Mark offered to take Laura for a while. She went gladly to him, he hoisted her onto his shoulders, they strolled through the crowd. Parked on the edges of the blocked-off streets were the cars driven by my ilk, the adventurous-sounding vehicles that denote the settled life: Outback, Odyssey, Caravan.

When Mark came back, he was shocked. "I had *no idea*," he said, "how much people stare at her! It was totally weird!"

I told Theresa the story later, and said, "See? What did I tell you?"

"I believe you that it happens," she said. "But I just don't see it as much as you do."

Laura's distinctive features had come into focus for most, and so we were noticed. It was a matter of mild contention, between Theresa and me, as to how much this happened, and how much it mattered. Laura didn't create the stir she did in the early days, with her oxygen tank and nose tube, and in our usual haunts (bookstore, coffee shop, fly shop, library), she was ordinary and known. But on the street, she usually got a second glance. I assembled an unofficial taxonomy of stares: *sympathetic, furtive, appraising, speculative, quizzical, hostile, enthusiastic, uncomfortable, friendly, knowing.* But more than anything, I noticed the way time stopped, the transfixed seconds before the flinch. As if we lived in a world of birders, and Laura were a shadow on a branch.

It is the pause she was born to, as doctors ticked off infant field marks, arched palate and epicanthal fold; it continued, for two weeks, as Theresa and I inhabited a trance of our own, gazing at an infant's closed eyes, while her chromosomes were counted in a Portland lab. Under the microscope the trisomy appeared, the ultimate field mark, the third dot dividing her from the rest. It was, in the language of field guides, "diagnostic." As a sometime birder, I know that satisfaction. You look carefully, and then it really is a grosbeak, or a black-and-blue warbler. But the fascination is deepest, the pleasure most intense, for the rare birds. For the accidental, the stray, the Asian migrant, paddling among the regular ducks, as if it belonged there. Something at home, yet out of place.

Tragedy and Expectation

That summer, Laura began attending a largish preschool near the university. She was two and a half years old, and kindergarten, though only a speck on the horizon, was close enough to plan for. If Laura was, as we hoped, to be included in a "regular" classroom, she would need to begin spending time with kids her age.

She cried when I dropped her off, at first. But she soon got used to the routine. I signed her in each morning, dropped off Ellie at her soccer camp, went off to write. After lunchtime, I'd pick Laura up; the daycare was quiet, the full-day kids asleep or drowsing on their blankets, afloat on peaceful, nauseating swells of Enya, and Laura would be coloring at a table or reading. I'd tiptoe in and Laura would turn, see me, and light up with a gigantic grin of recognition. I'd step over the sleepers and pick her up in a big hug. Then we'd go across campus to watch Ellie from the bleachers above the field. She was easy to pick out from a distance, her red jersey flopping around her legs as she sprinted for the ball.

We had tried lots of things with Ellie—hockey, modern dance, soccer—but soccer was the one she'd taken to, the one she played as if she'd always known how. Her passes were precise, her dribbling exact. This gave me inordinate satisfaction, though sometimes I found myself greedy, wanting her to be more aggressive, to cut through and score. One of the low points of my life as a father came a few years later, during one of her games, when I bellowed at her across the field to get open: "Give her a target!" Instantly, by her stricken stare, by the turned heads of other parents, I was convicted. It was the tone, the way I said it. I realized: Oh. I'm *that* asshole.

In raising both Ellie and Laura, in thinking about daycare and sports, friendships and kindergarten, the central question has always been the same: What can we reasonably expect? But in Laura's case, the question *What can we expect from Laura* is forever tangled with the other question, *What can you expect from a child with Down syndrome?*

In the beginning, when Laura was diagnosed, I had no idea. But beneath my ignorance were equations I could neither make explicit nor escape:

> *Laura = Down syndrome*
> *Down syndrome = abnormality*
> *abnormality = unhappiness*

Two and a half years later, the equations no longer held. Their terms were not the simple, unyielding variables I thought they were, so the equivalences failed. When I was unhappy, it was for the old reasons: insomnia, depression. My genome, my history, not hers. There were stresses with Laura, as with Ellie. But my daughters rescued me from unhappiness every day, in little things, in laughter and hugs and deft passes and new skills mastered, and they were part of the flexible, evolving structure in which happiness could occur. We were all part of it, a family, something lucky and difficult and irreplaceable.

Later in the summer, Laura was moved up to a class with kids her age. Because she was so small, I worried about her being picked on, but she seemed to be doing well. She did have a problem with one kid, but we found out only after the fact, on the day Laura dealt with it herself.

As it was explained to me later, the boy had been teasing her on the playground. It was teasing only, they said, nothing physical. But after lunch, when the full-day kids had already begun their naps, Laura went to the sink and filled a pitcher with water. Then she walked over to the sleeping boy and emptied it on his head.

— ◆ —

What *can* you expect, from a child with Down syndrome?

We have two basic answers. Both take the form of a story, and both will be familiar to most. In the first kind of story, a child is born; her parents are given a shocking diagnosis; the child grows, faces difficulties—some medical—but eventually takes his or her place in the family, and in the community. In the second kind of story, the child's arrival is a tragedy; the family is destroyed, siblings' lives eclipsed or ruined. In some versions, the community is harmed as well.

This was, of course, the irreconcilable pair of stories I faced, when Laura was born. Either Laura was a defect, or a child. Either we had the beginnings of a tragedy, or a story that could bring us joy. Two and a half years later, as I read my way through the open maze of the library stacks, I had a different perspective on this doubleness: whether the stories were hopeful or tragic, they seemed utterly distinct from Laura. I did not read them to learn what Laura's life might be.

There was no shortage of hopeful stories. There were the memoirs: *Life as We Know It, Expecting Adam, Matthew.* There were newspaper features about children who'd overcome difficulties, medical and otherwise, and were now thriving in school, or living on their own. There were articles and blogs by moms, dads, and siblings, and autobiographical writings by people with Down syndrome themselves: Chris Burke, Mia Peterson, Nigel Hunt. In general, these writings emphasized the person over the diagnosis, and told what was—despite difficulties—a happy story.

But there were tragedies too. In the textbook *Principles of Genetics* (2003), for example, a description of Down syndrome segues into predicted ruin:

> After five years of marriage, Michael and Carole decided
> that they were ready to begin their family. Carole soon
> became pregnant, and she and Michael eagerly awaited

the birth of their baby. It was a normal pregnancy and a
normal delivery. When their baby boy was born, however,
they knew immediately that something was wrong. The
child was lethargic and had poor muscle tone. His head
was short and very flat at the back; the eyes had a slanted appearance, and the irises had speckles around the
edges; the nose had a low bridge and the tongue tended
to protrude. These and other abnormalities all pointed
to one conclusion: The baby boy had Down syndrome.
Examination of the baby's cells showed that he had 47 instead of 46 chromosomes. The extra chromosome was the
smallest chromosome, chromosome number 21. The diagnosis was confirmed.

The textbook's authors clearly intend to show "the human side" of
genetics. But Michael and Carole do not react in believable ways. Most
parent narratives describe a life-destroying shock. People get drunk,
they weep, they see the wasteland of all their hopes. By these standards,
Michael and Carole are weirdly calm. Even weirder: although they have
clearly memorized most of the phenotypic features of Down syndrome,
although their eager anticipation is clearly focused on a normal child,
they have not bothered to test. (I am still trying to figure out what that
first postpartum conversation sounded like: "Honey, something is
wrong! The eyes appear to be somewhat slanted, and the tongue tends
to protrude. And are those Brushfield spots I detect?")

The story ends here. The boy is unnamed. If his parents, like most,
get over their affect-free state and come to accept him, we do not hear
it. If his lethargy fades, if he eventually learns to read and write, if he is
sick or healthy or sick first and healthy later, we don't know. In place of
story, we have a prediction:

> . . . the boy will grow up to be seriously retarded and will
> have a 1500 percent increased risk for developing leuke-
> mia. If he survives to adulthood, he will almost certainly

develop early-onset Alzheimer's disease. All of these problems develop because of the extra dose of genetic material
he carries.

This is a textbook. Future doctors read it. If they want to learn that
people with Down syndrome can have fulfilling lives, they will have to
rent old episodes of *Life Goes On*, then find a VHS player to watch them
on. They might consider shopping at the Arc, which runs thrift stores
to help intellectually disabled adults.

I was beginning to understand that the two narratives—hope and
tragedy—could not be reconciled. It was not just that they were starkly
different. It was that they were not talking about the same thing. One
kind of story was about an actual individual. It described that individual's trajectory through a particular time and in a particular place.
The tragedy, though, was typically a projection: it imagined what an
individual's story *might* be like.

At the heart of this projection was the list of diagnostic features.
The tragedy is the list in motion: if the list is a snapshot, the tragedy is
a movie. But then, if a child is only the sum of medical abnormalities—
*retardation, heart defect, intestinal atresia, obesity, torticollis, hypoto-
nia, leukemia, early-onset dementia, shortened life expectancy*—then
what story, but a tragedy, could she possibly have?

Here, for perspective, are three popular tragedies:

OEDIPUS REX: You accidentally sleep with your mom, and then
also accidentally kill your dad, because you tried to avoid a prophecy
that those exact things would happen. You feel bad, so you gouge your
eyes out. Children laugh at you. On the plus side, you are somewhat
wiser.

HAMLET: You have problems with prioritizing and time management,
a tendency to mope, and difficulty relating to women. In general, others annoy you. You are also behind schedule on the revenge killing of

your uncle, who is sleeping with your mom after having poisoned your dad, who periodically appears in ghostly form, asking you to hurry. You procrastinate. The kingdom is lost. Most of the main characters die, including you.

KING LEAR: Your retirement plan: divide your kingdom among your three daughters, according to their claims of love; then depend on their charity. One daughter (Cordelia: genuine, loving) refuses to speak. The remaining two (Regan, Goneril) tell the expected lies. You give them everything and disinherit the loving one, saying, more or less, "Thy truth be thy dower, beeyotch!" Betrayals and blindings follow—again, with the eyes—and after a storm described on The Weather Channel as "a doozy," you return, just in the nick of time, to save the good daughter from being hanged. Not! Then you die of heartbreak.

It's peculiar, even perverse, but when I think of Cordelia, I imagine her with Down syndrome.

She is, like so many, the youngest child. She is defined, not by speech, but by its absence. And she challenges us as Down syndrome does. She asks us about the nature of parental love, and to what extent that love is, or *can* be, unconditional. She asks what love has to do with language: "Love, and be silent," she says; "my love's / More richer than my tongue." She speaks, significantly, to herself; her most eloquent speeches are asides, murmurs that go unheard. In the realm of the court, she is an outsider.

Lear is soon cast out as well. Regan and Goneril steadily humiliate him, reducing his retinue of servants, banning him from the castles he bequeathed. Ranting against this generational betrayal, he curses Goneril with an end to generation:

> *Nature, hear! Dear goddess, hear!*
> *Suspend thy purpose, if thou didst intend*
> *To make this creature fruitful!*

But there is, he continues, a fate worse than infertility. If she should bear a child, he says, "let it be a thwart, disnatured torment to her." He curses her, in other words, with a birth defect: only a monster can equal a monstrous ingratitude. In neither case, Lear implies, can love be possible.

Down syndrome is not inherently tragic, but the questions raised by prenatal diagnosis are tragic in nature. Tragedy involves family, and the meaning of the links between generations. It is never far from the moral, or the mortal. Its characters live at the limits of language, with the unspeakable and unspoken. They are confronted, often, with muddy prophecies—partial information, cryptic utterances, blurry futures, a fate seen through frosted glass.

But tragedy is not about fate, exactly. It is about what, paradoxically, is fated *yet avoidable*. It is a sequence of events that is inexorable, and yet which—with the crucial fact, the single drop of wisdom—might also be averted. For those who believe Down syndrome leads inevitably to misery, prenatal diagnosis provides the essential knowledge, the prophecy to be heeded. The very availability of this knowledge, the fact that misery could have been averted, makes the resulting situation seem *more* tragic. A normal child could have been born instead.

If a woman is facing the difficult question of whether to continue a pregnancy with an affected fetus, and if she has not already made up her mind before the test, then what sort of knowledge is appropriate? How should Down syndrome be imagined? To talk about a representative person with the syndrome denies the syndrome's variability. To list every possible defect exaggerates the condition's seriousness. None of these set the condition in context. None describe what an ordinary life might be like; none hold out the possibility of happiness, except as a footnote. As such, the normal ways of describing the syndrome fall short of the ideal of "nondirectiveness" that genetic counselors seek to live up to—that is, an accurate description that both clarifies the situation, yet preserves the autonomy of the woman making the decision. A description that frames unanswerable questions: What will life be like? Will happiness be possible?

Strictly speaking, that knowledge can only be had with experience. But what can be provided are lives accurately imagined: a realistic vision of risk, and an equally realistic vision of possibility. Ideally, the woman will have a sensitive, informed, unbiased genetic counselor, who will guide her through the realities, and offer to put her in touch with families who have lived with the condition. Such an approach, as the disability rights theorist and feminist Adrienne Asch points out, will *increase* choice, not limit it: many descriptions simply assume a child with Down syndrome is a burden, a portrayal both incorrect and paternalistic. If women are grown-up enough to control their own reproduction, they are grown-up enough to deal with *all* the realities of the condition, including the medical risks, available community resources, and the benefits amply witnessed by parents. A mistaken portrait helps no one.

July 2003

Laura is asleep at last. I have two hours to write. I shouldn't let her nap, but it's the end of the week, she's exhausted, I'm exhausted, I'll let her watch TV later. Maybe she'll sleep through the night, if she goes to sleep by eleven. Though I doubt it.

She's heavier. Twisting and bending over, laying her in the crib, I feel the shift in weight, like a human gyroscope. I settle her down, raise the rail, and drape the quilt over the crib to keep the sun out. The quilt slides to the floor. I reposition it, more evenly this time, and it collapses inward. She stirs. I lift its soft folds away from her, carefully, the way you'd lift a bandage from a wound, and I set it on the floor and tiptoe out. I go downstairs and out to the shed and find a couple of spring clamps. I go back upstairs and clamp the quilt in place above her head, and the moment's satisfaction is tiny but real, like being shipwrecked, but finding a really big piece of wood to hang on to. In the universe right next to ours, we already have curtains on the window above Laura's bed. In that universe I am punctual with self-administered deadlines, and radiant with a serene acceptance of the undone. But I'm living here, in the La Brea tar pits of the unfinished. I have an hour and forty-five minutes to write. I go downstairs to fix lunch.

Ellie is at the dining room table, coloring an elaborate geometric pattern. It dumbfounds me, like everything she does: I was a slob, I colored over the lines. She is obsessive/intense, like me, but organized, not like me. I ask her if she wants some ramen for lunch and she says, "Yes, Dad!" I start boiling a pan of water. I get a ten-cent package of beef-flavored dried ramen and tear the plastic open. It looks like freeze-dried tissue: dense but light, ivory-colored, its strands wavy and parallel. I drop it in the boiling water. I tear open the foil packet and shake the powder into the water, where it foams up its beefy essence, then disperses. Green flecks churning in the water, the strands of ramen coming apart. I throw away the foil packet and the plastic wrapper. I get out bowls. I dish out ramen for both of us and we eat and I tell her that her coloring looks great and she says, "Thanks!" I have an hour and fifteen minutes to write.

I let Laura sleep too long, I write a little bit, Ellie goes off to play with a friend. I hear Laura waking up and go upstairs. I change her diaper (soaked, sagging, puffy) and wipe the sweat from her face and get her a snack. I clown around to wake her up. She gets down from her booster seat and goes to the piano.

For Laura the piano is a texture, a toy, a way to be like Ellie: now and then, she'll reach up and turn the pages of Ellie's music, as if she were sight-reading. But playing, she looks down at the keys the way you'd look at a moving stream. She presses out mild, white-key dissonances with the gathered tips of her fingers. She angles her wrists like a baker, as if the articulated levers, felt-tipped hammers, and tripled strings were so much bread dough.

I stand behind her, a little bored. I can't read the new *Harper's*, or tie flies, since she could fall from the piano bench. So I reach around her, plink out one measure of a Two-Part Invention, last vestige of the lessons I quit in high school. She seizes my right hand and flings it away. I play the next measure, teasing her a little, and she says "DAAAAA!" Laughing, as she yells. She's copying Ellie. When Ellie sits down after school and asks for Apple Jacks, and I bring her an enormous mixing bowl, then apologize, and bring a shot glass, then bring a regular bowl with Apple Jacks and milk but no spoon, then go out and come back with a shovel, saying, "Robot bring you spoon!"—then Ellie screams, "Daaaad!" It gets us through the day.

DAAAA has been Laura's all-purpose syllable for quite some time, inflected to mean, variously, *Dad, yes, happy,* and so on; it's been here since before her signing began to take off, and I like to think of *DAAAA* as a cornerstone of whatever language she might acquire, a conceit both egotistical and true. She grabs my hand again and flings it away.

People with Down syndrome are supposed to be "musical." But Ellie has always been the musician in the family. She loved the piano from an early age, giving me hope that for her, piano practice might be something other than a suburban penance. Laura likes music just fine, but she has no special affinity or talent for it, chromosomal or otherwise. Also unlike Ellie, she doesn't put up with the clinically depressed alt-country lullabies that filled Ellie's childhood bedtimes, the doleful songs by John Hiatt and Steve Earle and Lucinda Williams. Laura wants "Five Little Monkeys," like a normal kid.

That spring, their differing tastes in music became an issue. In the bright yellow Mazda we'd bought in May, we had a CD player, a novelty for us. (Even in 2003, most of our music was still on cassette tapes.) Ellie and Laura regularly fought over what to listen to. Ellie wanted Coldplay or U2 or The Beatles. Laura wanted the *Toddler Favorites* CD, with "Twinkle, Twinkle," "Five Little Monkeys," and all the others. The rest of us had had it with *Toddler Favorites.* The singer gave us the willies: she sounded like a preschool teacher on crank. We had memorized every last guitar fill and inflection of her voice, plus the irritatingly cute, off-key kids joining in on half the songs, and we were ready to throw it away, but we put it on, because listening to *Toddler Favorites* is not half as bad as trying to listen to U2 while Laura *asks* for *Toddler Favorites*. In a rare success, Ellie later taught Laura to scream "ATHO ATHO" to the chorus of "Vertigo," but there are only so many times you can hear *that* song, especially when the iPod commercials are in heavy rotation on TV.

Not that we would see the iPod commercials, when Laura was watching the second Harry Potter movie.

Laura never asked for the CD in words others would recognize, but her wishes were unmistakable all the same. I thought of my old days teaching argumentation to college students, the fine points of structure and syntax and word choice and organization, and it occurred to me that inside the yellow car, these conventions were irrelevant. Persistence was what mattered. Laura had no syntax, hardly even a spoken word, and yet she consistently won.

That August, we flew back East. We took the redeye to Durham, our previous hometown. We stayed with friends there, ate at Bullock's Barbeque, felt the paralyzing humidity we'd forgotten, saw the gaping hole where the dowdy old mall had been. Our friends took us, in an archaeology-of-the-immediate kind of way, to the new mall, with its fanatically padded children's play area, gigantic food court, and faux-European cobblestoney pedestrian streets. Ellie goggled at the Mac Store: she loves gadgets more than I do. Laura saw her first in-theater movie, *Finding Nemo*, which excited and terrified her: she kept running up the aisle of the empty theater to Theresa, gesturing at the screen, signing *fish*, saying something that sounded like *whale*.

After two days, we drove south to Myrtle Beach to meet Theresa's family—her sisters, brother, mother, and all of Ellie and Laura's cousins. By then, Laura's sleep schedule was atomized, destroyed. She inhabited the time zones of several continents, none of them ours. She napped from five in the afternoon until seven in the evening, stayed up till one, fell asleep, woke up in the middle of the night for an hour, went back to sleep, slept in till eleven. She'd been clinging to Theresa, mainlining Mom for hours on end—the novelty of it, having Mom all day, nothing but Mom, Mom in the morning and Mom at night, Mom to herself while Dad surf-fished and Ellie screamed in the waves with her cousins. One night, at eleven, when Laura was clearly just getting revved up for another two and a half hours of play, I said, "Here, I'll take her." We drove to the Wal-Mart Supercenter.

The parking lot was disorientingly huge. Football fields. Proving grounds. I drove the rented Suzuki across the lane lines, parked near the entrance. Inside, I let Laura rifle through sweatpants and T-shirts on their hangers. We played peekaboo. I picked out a shirt for three dollars, another for four. "This way, Laura," I said, "this way," the distance like elastic between us. I backed away, beckoning, keeping her in sight. I could see her deciding whether to follow, then smiling, rushing towards me, hands already up.

We could have been five thousand feet underground, after the end of civilization. That several miles away, past roadside culverts, palm trees with browning fronds, and billboards advertising lookalike superstars, Theresa was back with Susie at the vacation condo, surfing through eighty channels of cable, I did not doubt, but that life seemed a shadow.

"Mum mum," said Laura, and I said, brightly, "Later! We'll see her later!" I did our made-up sign for *later*, two index fingers indicating an event stage right. As if she'd asked for directions, and I'd said, "No, the place you want is two doors down." Later.

We circumnavigated the store. She signed *up*, and I lifted her into the cart. We played the game Ellie and I played, years ago: I shove the cart away from me, let it coast, and then look around distracted, saying, "Where's Laura? Where is she?" Then I see her, run after, and save her, just before the cart plows into the air fresheners.

She signed *eat*. We found the cafeteria, about an eighth of a mile away. It was closed. She saw the Formica, stainless steel, and plastic, and signed *French fries*—her instinct for junk food is unerring—but the registers were unattended. "No, Laura," I said. "It's closed now." She signed *French fries*. I said: "Let's find something else! How about apple?" She shook her head. "Avocado?" She signed *down*. I set her down. She led me forward, hand closed around my index finger, in her cheerful half-run, half-stumble, head down, charging forward. We walked past Intimates, Baby, Men's Apparel, Sporting Goods, Magazines, and soon we were in the supermarket section, itself bigger than any supermarket in our hometown.

Laura ran ahead; I followed. She signed, again, *French fry, French fry*. "No, Laura," I said. "No, it's closed." *French fry!* she signed, more definite. I shook my head. We were in the frozen foods section. She pointed, exasperated, at the glass door: behind it were boxes and boxes of Ore-Ida frozen deep-fried potato products: Tater Tots, steak fries, crinkle cut fries, the pictures magnified, glistening with fat. *French fries*.

We paid and left. It was twelve-thirty in the morning. The air was humid, and in the parking lot, light pooled at the base of each tower. I set Laura in her car seat, buckled her in, loaded up the bag of vacation groceries: Cokes, Oreos, milk, cereal, chips. I opened the bag of Cheetos we'd bought in line, handed it backwards as we pulled away, felt her tug it from my hand. By the time we got back to the condo, her face was completely orange.

John Langdon Down

We flew home, tired and restored. Theresa settled into an autumn of grants, committee work, and teaching, though *settling* does not quite describe the chaos of an assistant professor's life, as her tenure decision nears. Ellie began the second grade at Jefferson School. Her main subjects seemed to be Reading, Math, and Watershed Science. Her class tromped out to the creek behind the school to see what lived there. There were frogs, suckers, cutthroat trout. It was good to be home.

On Thursday afternoons, we'd drive to Linda Hansen's house for Ellie's piano lesson. There was a canoe hanging above the garage, a Subaru parked in front. The house was in a neighborhood north of the university, where the tidy grid of streets (presidents, crossed with numbers) yields to winding streets named for trees. There were ranch houses, shaded by Douglas firs. Ellie loved Linda; her house was a refuge, as piano was a refuge for Ellie, and they hit it off in the way you always hope your kid and her piano teacher will. I liked sitting with Laura on my lap, in an end-of-the-week good tired, listening to Ellie play, and seeing her light up at Linda's affectionate praise.

When Ellie was at school, Laura and I would meet Theresa for lunch. We'd pick her up and drive away from campus, deciding where to eat. Laura, sensing an opening, would sign furiously for FRIES in the back, and we would cave and say "sure" and wind up at the same Wendy's we'd gone to when she was eating through a tube in her nose. We'd spread the fries on her tray to cool, saying and signing *hot*—in the sign, the hand flicks backwards, from an imaginary burn—and Laura would say "ah" and then blow on the fries to cool them. She ate them one by one, dipping each one in a puddle of ketchup.

Sometimes I talked about the book I was writing. I'd been reading about John Langdon Down, learning exciting new facts about the Royal Earlswood Asylum for Idiots, where Down lived, worked, and discovered the patients who would later bear his name. Eventually Theresa would say something like, "You know, it might be time to hold off on the research for a while," or "You know, we really need to think about getting you some more childcare." After lunch, we'd drop her at the back entrance to the College of Pharmacy and head home. Then I'd put on Elmo and scribble notes on colored cards.

Many parents raise children with Down syndrome without ever knowing a thing about John Langdon Down. It's not *necessary* to know the history of Down syndrome, in the way that it might be necessary, say, to know how to deal with crankiness in a child of few words, or how to put in a feeding tube. But for me, as a writer, a father, and a son, the history *was* necessary. I had come to see that we inherit misunderstanding, that the misunderstanding falls into patterns, and that the patterns are imaginative responses to contradiction. Whether we say *a child first* or *a Down syndrome child*, whether we reduce children to lists or tell stories to which the list is a footnote, whether we speak with hope or the conviction of tragedy, we are always grappling with the doubleness of child and condition. Every pattern responds to the fact of children who seem radically different, yet human too.

It's tempting to think of this doubleness as recent. To say, for example, that it results from an incomplete metamorphosis. That once upon a time, things were bad, and now things are better, but not all the way better; that we are stuck between an old idea of tragedy, and a new idea of hope. But I don't think this is true. The discovery of the forty-seventh chromosome is comparatively new, but the way we talk about Down syndrome is very old.

John Langdon Down is usually described as the condition's discoverer, as if the chromosome were an exotic continent, and he were the first explorer to reach it. But the children existed before they were discovered; what changed, after Down, was the way they were known. Like other explorers, Down both named and described the territory he found, and though we have rejected the name he chose, the terms of his description are still with us. Our patterns begin with him.

It was inevitable that the syndrome would be discovered: that with the rise of the asylum in Great Britain, people with trisomy 21 would be lifted from the invisibility of almshouses and attics and gathered in groups, that their affinities would be noticed, then translated into diagnosis. It was not inevitable, however, that they would be named "Mongolian idiots." That phrase—brilliant, memorable, wrong—was Down's invention. It lasted for decades, and it may have had its genesis in his chance meeting with an intellectually disabled girl.

He was eighteen at the time. To hear him tell it, that encounter shaped his future. Late in his life, at the opening of a new wing at Normansfield—the private, for-profit asylum he founded at the age of forty-one—he told the story:

> In a remote part of the country on an alfresco picnic . . .
> driven by stress of weather into a cottage on the coast, I
> was brought into contact with a feeble minded girl, who
> waited on our party and for whom the question haunted
> me—could nothing for her be done? I had then not entered
> on a medical student's career, but ever and anon the
> remembrance of that hapless girl presented itself to me
> and I longed to do something for her kind.

Perhaps this really was the lightning strike, the key experience, that sparked Down on his rise to fame and wealth. It is hard to say. At eighteen, Down seemed destined to a modest future as a shopkeeper. He'd been taken out of school four years before, to work beneath his father and older brother in the family store, a combined grocery and pharmacy. (He had been born in an upstairs room.) According to his biographer, O. Conor Ward, Down enjoyed concocting new medicines and toiletries (including Down's Celebrated Lavender Water, Down's Rose Dentifrice, and Down's Vaseline Pomade), but otherwise despised the shop. In 1853, within weeks of his father's death, he left to become a doctor.

As a medical student at London Hospital, Down took a heavier-than-usual courseload, won awards in every subject, completed his apothecary's training, took electives at the University of London, volunteered among the poor, and finished almost a year early. Upon graduation, he began a six-month obstetrics appointment at the hospital; it was extended for three years. Only then, when a scandal at the Royal Earlswood Asylum for Idiots resulted in an vacancy there, did Down begin his life of ministering to the people who were, as a matter of diagnosis, referred to as *idiots*. It had been twelve years since his encounter with "the feeble minded girl."

Whether the girl set him on his path, or whether he was scoring chance with the soundtrack of destiny, is impossible to know. For me, what rings true is the element of surprise. The syndrome does not enter a life gradually. You go on a picnic, and your life changes. You are brought into contact, and haunted thereafter.

As David Wright points out in his history of Earlswood Asylum, *Mental Disability in Victorian England: The Earlswood Asylum, 1847–1901*, there are two public versions of Down. In one, he is, in his biographer's phrase, "a caring pioneer"; in another, he is a racist, self-serving opportunist. In Wright's balanced and thoughtful account, there is plenty of evidence for both positions. His work at Earlswood cannot be reduced to the profit motive. Earlswood was a charitable institution, and Down's reforms were too imaginative and labor intensive to have been driven by greed. And yet his career was shaped less by charity than by entrepreneurship: he left Earlswood after a minor scandal, when he was found to be looking after private patients off the books, and soon after leaving Earlswood, he opened Normansfield, a for-profit institution for children of the wealthy. As for his ideas of "idiocy," he often manifests a genuine kindness, a racial view liberal for his time, and a respect for possibility and development; and yet, by the terms of his published classification, his "Mongolian idiots" were a lesser kind of human being. His truest legacy is contradiction.

When he took over at Earlswood, Down had no professional experience with what was then called "idiocy." The asylum had been founded seven years before with inspirational words of uplift and moral instruction, but these fine intentions had run aground on filthy bedsheets, financial mismanagement, and medical neglect. Down had panicky second thoughts after accepting the post, but his appointment at Earlswood is the reason we still say his name. It was the first asylum in England built exclusively for "idiots"; it probably held the nation's first significant gathering of people with trisomy 21. For a young, ambitious doctor, they were a pattern waiting to be recognized.

When I first read "Observations on an Ethnic Classification of Idiots"— the short paper in which Down unveiled his diagnosis—I was surprised to find an oft-repeated word: *family*. It is a touchstone idea for Down. It is his term for the species ("the great human family"); for race ("the great Caucasian family," "the great Mongolian family"); and for his patients, whom he referred to as "family members."

Down's use of the word reflects the problem he faced. His patients did not resemble their parents. More significantly, to Down, they did not even seem to belong to their parents' *race*. They had been born to Caucasians, but had "Mongolian" features. "It is difficult to realise," wrote Down about one of his trisomic patients, "that he is the child of Europeans." And yet they did resemble each other: "When placed side by side," Down writes, "it is difficult to believe that the specimens compared are not children of the same parents." "Difficult to realise," "difficult to believe": you can sense the man's struggle with the questions his "specimens" raised. They did not seem to belong anywhere. They were literally unfamiliar.

Down, as we know, solved his puzzle in terms of race. From the "great Mongolian family," and the literal families of his patients, he created a new family of "Mongolian idiots," who belonged to neither and both. That family, according to Down, was only one of several. There were idiots, Down claimed, of "the Ethiopian variety"; "types of the family which people the South Sea Islands"; and "analogues of the people who . . . originally inhabited the American Continent." All, in Down's view, had suffered from "degeneration" before birth. Taken together, they constituted a system, an ethnic classification. (Down acknowledges the fact that most of his idiots are Caucasian, but does not dwell on the point.)

To formulate his theory, Down had to assume two ideas today's biologists reject. The first is that "race" has a simple, definite meaning: that humankind can be divided into five tidy, continent-sized boxes, each labeled "Mongol," "African," and so on. Though this *popular* understanding still endures, most biologists see race as a fiction. Human differences are real, but they are too complex to sort into boxes: there is as much variation *within* the entire continent of Africa, where our species originated, as within the species as a whole.

The second assumption, of course, was that the races could be ranked. Down does not say so explicitly, but at the same time his theory leaves little doubt. He could not believe his patients had suffered "degeneration" from a white ideal, and at the same time hold that all races were equal. Though Down, as is often pointed out, was liberal for his time—he opposed slavery, and unlike some scientists of his day, believed all human beings had a common descent—he also clearly felt that some human beings were more equal than others. A hierarchy of races, with Caucasians at the top, underpins his theory.

It would be easy to dismiss Down as a racist. That's what I thought he was, at first. But as several writers have pointed out, Down's racism is not so simple. In the final paragraph of his "Observations," he springs from his ethnic classification to a speculation on human unity: if a child can change its racial profile in utero, Down reasoned, then the boundaries between races are indefinite. "Degeneracy," therefore, implied "the unity of the human species." Having carefully partitioned humanity into groups, Down uses "Mongolian idiocy" to prove that the groups are porous. It is a strange, paradoxical turn.

To read the "Observations" is a strange experience. On the one hand, Down solemnly insists on the importance of consistency and objectivity and of framing a "natural system"—one true to the facts— as opposed to one that is "artificial." And yet the paper itself is far from systematic. He proposes a system to which, he admits, most of his patients do not belong. His classification describes five ethnic types, but he focuses only on one. He rambles, digresses, delivers asides on treatment, therapy, personality traits, human descent. He mentions that his theory might be useful in defending physicians from malpractice: if the condition is congenital, then anxious parents cannot, for example, blame a nurse for an opium overdose, or the physician for a forceps delivery gone wrong.

Stranger yet is Down's incuriosity about the question of cause. He hardly addresses the obvious question: *how* did this happen? Given the enormity of his claim—that *like* could beget *unlike*, that parents of Race A could produce children with features of Race B, and that, moreover, all human beings had a common ancestor—you might think he would explore the question. But beyond a speculation that the condition is sparked by tuberculosis, Down has little to say. In a sort of verbal shrug, Down writes, "Here, however, we have examples of retrogression, or, at all events, of departure from one type and the assumption of the characteristics of another." Retrogression? Departure? Whatever it was, "degeneration" could account for it: "so frequently are these characters presented," Down writes, "that there can be no doubt that these ethnic features are the result of degeneration."

Given Down's research, and his other publications, the absence of evidence is striking. Down collected data for eight years. In critiquing the work of other scientists, he can be exacting and skeptical, attentive to statistical and logical errors. And yet with "Mongolian idiocy," and with Down's ethnic classifications in general, his standards all but disappear. He would be the first of many. Down syndrome, like the North Pole, causes compass needles to spin: and more than one researcher has found himself atop his destination, mystified and lost.

Reading Down's slim, collected writings, I remembered the days after Laura arrived. Everything was questioned; everything I lived by was suddenly, radically strange. What did *family* mean now? What would our family be like, and what did that have to do with the family I came from? Being "half" white and "half" Japanese: what did that mean, exactly? I'd written poetry about that mixed inheritance, but day to day, I didn't think about it much. I lived it from the inside out; beneath the unconscious dailiness of identity was a pride in my heritage. I did not live by halves. And yet, in the appearance of my second daughter, these categories meant something else. In those early weeks, as Laura's diagnosis was confirmed, and as my mother and I fell out over an old, erroneous label, this sense of strangeness persisted. It was not enough to know that Down was wrong. We seemed haunted by the history, pervaded by it, and until I understood the history I could not be entirely free.

Our lives seemed an echo chamber for the past: a nineteenth-century mistake was audible in our twenty-first-century lives. Now, two and a half years later, those echoes reechoed, multiplied by distance. What I'd faced as a father, I faced again as a writer. Family, ethnicity, inheritance, disability, belonging . . . in Down's little paper, the machine of identity seemed shattered and reassembled into a machine of misunderstanding. Everything in Down's paper seemed familiar and unfamiliar at once. But that was how his "idiots" seemed to him, and, in a very different way, that was how Laura first seemed to us. She had arrived in our family, but she was radically unfamiliar. *A child first.*

That fall, I began building Ellie a bed. She'd long since outgrown the crib mattress she'd slept on when our bedrooms were downstairs, and the futon she was using seemed makeshift somehow. We'd been moved in upstairs for a while, but it still felt like we were camping, half the time.

At first, the bed was supposed to be a simple platform nailed together from CDX plywood. Several sheets of graph paper later, the bed had acquired a solid ash headboard with a built-in bookshelf and a footboard with red oak panels striped by walnut inlays. I didn't finish it until March. Ellie helped sand the parts, wearing outsized safety glasses and ear protection and gloves to dampen the sander's vibrations. She helped buff the wax too, and handed me hardware when I bolted the rails to the headboard and footboard. Years later, she's still using the bed, and when I think back about building it for her, I am glad I stopped reading about John Langdon Down for a while.

The upstairs renovation, over two years after I'd started, was all but complete. The bathroom only lacked a door, but I used this to my advantage. Laura was then at the beginning of our epic journey towards successful use of the potty, working towards the Grail of Toileting, and I was finding that what worked best, the positive reinforcement that kept Laura perched and happy, were the stuffed animals.

I would set Laura on the potty, and then, hidden in the adjacent bedroom, I would wing stuffed animals past the open doorway. We had about a bushel and a half, most left over from Laura's hospitalization—nothing attracts fluffy bunnies like a mortally sick child—and so, as she sat giggling, I would hurl them past the door, one at a time, the purple Princess Diana bear, the hippopotamus, the Gund bear, the zombielike, blue-eyed plastic dolls. Then, after a long pause, I would pick up the Tupperware moving container and heave the whole pile through the open door, which on the best days sent Laura into unstoppable giggles. She sometimes hunched her shoulders when she laughed, as if she were at the same time embarrassed, a little, at the silliness of it all.

October 2003

We're sitting at the dining room table, drawing. Laura bends her head close to the page, a pink eraser waggling beside her right ear. She scribbles, right to left, left to right, as if scrubbing a persistent stain, the lines shallow arcs like drafts of a horizon. She seizes a wad of pages, flips them over. She doesn't quite have the fine motor control to grasp and turn a single sheet, so the notebook fills in here and there: some pages dense and detailed, others blank, others marked with a single, hurried check.

She's discovered, on her own, how to hold a pencil. Another surprise: her grip is deft, coordinated, exact. It was a tiny relief, to see her writing—one less worry, on the long to-do list of inclusion.

I say, "Laura, can you draw a circle?" I whirl the pencil around, trying to make it fun. She obliges, the pencil point revolving like an electron. Each orbit overlaps the last, until a shell of traces surrounds a center. I praise her. I say, "Okay, try this one." I do a jagged line, an EKG, a ripsaw, a *W* that forgot to stop. She copies that too. I say, hopefully, "Laura, can you draw *A*?" I draw an *A*. She is losing interest. "Look, Laura," I say, "look! *A!*" But she's bored now, and the little voice tells me to leave it alone. I leave it alone. She returns to scribbling. Straight lines, left to right, right to left.

Writing mattered enough to Laura that she invented two signs for it. Both are obvious, intuitive, universal. In the first, she pats the carpet beside her: *Sit down next to me.* In the second, she mimes scribbling: fingertips to thumb, as in the sign *more,* but tilted downward, tracing ovals on an imaginary page. ("Do you want to write, Laura?" "Da." "Can you say write?" "Da"—which either means "yes, I can, but choose not to," or "duh," as in, "I *am* saying 'write.'")

I decide to end the day's lesson. If she's imitating a circle now, that's already *O*; we'll get to *A* someday. I hand Laura the tin of pencils and crayons. She dumps them out, pats her thigh: *draw me a dog*. I draw the same bulbous caricature of Penny I used to draw for Ellie. She pats her thigh again. "You draw it," I say, handing her the pencil. She tries to, tracing a careful oval for the head, stabbing two dots in place for eyes, then adding a little squib on the oval's end: the nose. The pencil moves slowly, as if a magnet were moving under the paper, trying to pull the point off course. As if she were tracing a line against the grain. But I'm happy. I say, "Dog, Laura, you drew a dog! Hooray!"

It only looks like a dog if you know the context. To anyone else, it's a vague oval, overwritten with scribbles. And yet—to me, at least— what's illegible is expressive. Every shape is a definition. The scribbles, unplaceable, unnamable, resist the boxes and blanks of expectation. It's a sentimental conceit, I know—she has no idea, yet, of the way the world furrows its brow over her—but knowing Laura, with her stubborn determination, I like to think of her refusing expectation, drawing whatever she wants.

Thinking this, I know that it *is* sentimental, that it's not that simple. I enforce the very expectations I resist. I, too, want her scrawl to morph into an alphabet anyone can read; I too, in describing her handwriting, want to trim her scribbles to neat Euclidean categories: line, circle, square. These categories are print beneath the signature, anonymous Helvetica beneath the beauty of an individual scrawl. She's blurred by my definitions.

We approximate each other. Laura, like Ellie before her, is trying to write our shapes and alphabet, and as with Ellie, I'm writing about it, interpreting the scribble as a fond and hopeful father. That Ellie was quicker to learn, and will learn more, has become less important to me than the fact of learning. It's enough for me, most days, that Laura's making progress. That there is a curve to plot, a line that resembles hope.

Minutes from Laura's six-month IFSP review, October 8, 2003. Recorded in the clear, slightly hurried print of Morning McCreary, Laura's Toddler Group teacher and new EI coordinator.

> **Cognitive:** sorting by color, size (big & little), kind – continue
> **Adaptive:** toileting, dressing – making progress – continue
> **Gross motor:** jumping, stairs w/handrail – stairs good progress
> > *tricycle – still need to adapt the pedals with blocks.
> **Fine motor:** work on open web space with coloring, stringing beads – can do the 1st step of stringing – continue w/ 2nd part.
> **Receptive language:** follow 3 step directions w/novel concepts. Understands in and on for prepositions. What & where for familiar.
> **Expressive:** imitate oral motor movements – met
> **PT** – needs general strengthening & balance activities.
> > Will add: walking on a balance beam standing on one leg, 3 sec.

November 2003

Laura sits on the carpet I have yet to replace, turning the cardboard pages of her favorite book: William Wegman's *One, Two, Three*. She says *du, twee,* pointing to mournful Weimaraners dressed in monks' robes, or gazing out, from a starkly lit dock, over a darkened lake. She signs as she talks, unfurling thumb, index, middle.

She is miming the act of reading: When she says *du*, drawing out the *u*, she is looking at six dogs. She slaps her thigh to sign *dog*. She pages backwards towards *one*. Though she looks like a tiny scholar in search of a citation—combing the stiff pages for a footnote, murmuring to herself, tracing the page with a forefinger—she does not yet, as far as I can tell, understand sequence and plot, even in the epic novel whose denouement is a row of ten snuggly puppies. You might as well say *two* as *three*, *du* as *twee*; you might as well say *twee* before *du*; you might as well blend them, as she does, playing with the sounds, saying *duuuuu-weeee*. Numbers are porous to her. They run, blur, absorb each other. They are not *hard*, in the way we believe quantities to be hard. She does not yet understand the metrics applied to her life so far, the blood pressures, milliliters, measurements against the norm.

And then I look down and see her looking at *seven*: a photograph of two dogs, cropped to show seven legs. The back legs are blurred. Laura is saying "duuuweee"—the number that stands for Number—but she is visibly counting, pointing to one dog leg, then the next. I've never seen this. The action has a deliberate quality, a shading of intention, that I find completely new. She counts each leg only once.

Every achievement has a history. Theresa spends hours reading to Laura, saying, "One, two, three! Laura, can you say, 'One, two, three'?" Laura says, "Duuuweee!" Ellie, in the car on the way to school, says, "Laura, can you say one, two, three?" And Laura, who would happily follow Ellie anywhere, even into language, tilts her head, smiles, and opens her hand like a numerical flower: thumb, index, middle, "duuu-weee!" Ellie imitates Theresa, Laura imitates Ellie, and from these replications and alterations grows a story, a living thread, a continuity vining across the calendar's divisions. The moment both includes and redeems the other moments that went to compose it, and so the days of an occasionally depressive stay-at-home dad, which can seem like a bad update of "The Rime of the Ancient Mariner"—a windless sea bobbing with diapers, half-eaten hot dogs, and broken Happy Meal toys, the air filled with Raffi and the ghost wails of dead parents—come to seem worthwhile. We're getting somewhere at last.

— ◆ —

Though John Langdon Down inhabited many roles—doctor, entrepreneur, asylum superintendent, devout family man—he was also a writer, and his writing is the reason we still remember him. If "Mongolian idiocy" lasted for decades, it's not just because Down's discovery was novel and real; it's because he translated that discovery into memorable language. With "Mongolian idiot," Down fused disparities into a vivid, surprising, and culturally resonant name.

That vividness has helped the name endure. Down's label has the punch of an image: he adds a face to an idea. The idea that imagistic writing is more powerful than other kinds remains a moldy truism among writing teachers—"show, don't tell"—but like all truisms, it has a grain of truth. A precise image, from Basho's haiku to Whitman's catalogs, has the power of a charm. The endurance of "Mongolian idiocy," however, owes as much to vagueness as precision. It's a precise blur, the face of a diagnosis. That blur is buried deep in Down's vision. Beneath his observations is a deep conviction that "Mongolian idiots" are essentially alike—a conviction expressed not only by the diagnosis itself, but by the way Down gives that diagnosis form.

When Down sets out to describe his "Mongolian idiots," he does something odd: he describes a single child. He does so, he says, because the children are so similar that one can stand for another: "They present such a close resemblance to one another in mental power, that I shall describe an idiot member of this racial division, selected from the large number that have fallen under my observation." With this stroke, Down *personifies* the syndrome, creating an Everyboy of idiocy, blurring child and diagnosis into a single, representative type. He then defines that type with a list, in which physical features (like "dirty-yellowish skin") are mixed with character attributes (like a tendency to imitation), notes on medical treatment, ideas about education, and fragmentary anecdotes. This is the pattern still common today.

But where did that pattern come from? Where did the writer get his form?

From the rhetoric of race. When Down chose to see his "idiots" in terms of race, he made use of the way race was understood.

The historian Nancy Stepan describes the rise of "race" as a product of Enlightenment science and colonial exploration. Classification and conquest went hand in hand: when the great systematizers of nature— Linnaeus and Buffon—needed data on non-European peoples, they had to depend on the information brought back by European explorers. "The tendency in science," writes Stepan, "was . . . to abstract general notions from the mass of information, ideas and suggestions about human groups collected by explorers—to transform travel literature into scientific text." What resulted, as Stepan writes, was a racial type: "an abstracted 'Negro' or 'Hottentot,'" who was compared (unfavorably) to "an abstracted and idealised European." That type was described with a list, in which physical qualities and presumed personality traits were freely mixed together. Skin color might be set beside "indolence"; hair texture, beside imagined sexual habits; eye-shape, beside a supposed tendency to steal.

This is the template for Down's diagnosis: he poured his "idiots" into a racial mold. But since he was also defining a medical condition, he included symptoms along with physical and mental characteristics. In this, the list's endless flexibility was useful. It bridged taxonomy and medicine; it helped him meld two systems of classification and throw in personality traits to boot. The result was as much character sketch as diagnosis: Down's unnamed boy, the child who stands for all children.

Though I can't be sure, I think this approach was psychologically useful to Down. Like many people today, Down had a profoundly conflicted attitude towards people with the syndrome. On the one hand, his patients were obviously weird and different. On the other hand, they were appealing in ordinary human ways. They were "amiable," educable, charming even in disobedience. I think Down's descriptive strategy reflects and resolves this conflict. The unnamed boy is human, but not individual. In fact, Down uses the singular pronoun only to describe physical features. When he begins to describe behaviors and personality traits, he switches to the plural "they."

We are still torn between perceptions of humanity and difference. We still assume people with Down syndrome are fundamentally like each other and unlike us. But to call this idea an "assumption" misses the mark. It is a deep, visceral reaction, like something the body thinks about another body. The way the eye sees another eye.

In 1966, a small conference met in London. Its occasion was the centennial of Down's "Observations on an Ethnic Classification of Idiots." Its proceedings, published in a slim volume a year later, were entitled *Mongolism: In Commemoration of Dr. John Langdon Haydon Down.*

A commemoration is an act as weighty as a statue, a gesture towards history. In context, it seems almost an act of denial. Down's legacy was in decline. His theory had been discarded long ago, and the term "Mongolism" was on its way out. Normansfield, the private asylum he founded after being forced out of Earlswood, would soon pass from his family. Though his sons Reginald and Percival, and then his grandson Norman, had overseen the asylum since his death, the institution would soon be investigated and closed. More and more, parents were assuming their children would go home with them.

But the conference chair—a neurologist named, improbably, Lord Brain—skirts unpleasant topics, choosing to remember Down as a scientist and a family man. He praises Down's innovations at Earlswood, but does not mention the scandal that precipitated his resignation. He notes Down's opposition to slavery, but avoids the ugly implications of "Mongolian idiocy." He lists Down's distinguished relatives: a bishop, an artist, a grand-niece who married John Maynard Keynes. We hear a great deal about genealogy, but nothing about degeneration. Perhaps this is because Lord Brain was married to Down's granddaughter Stella, and his brother-in-law, Norman Langdon-Down, was the current super-intendent of Normansfield. (Norman attended the conference, though he is not recorded as having spoken.)

But at the conference's conclusion, a Japanese geneticist, E. Matsunaga, questions the terms of memory. ("I am not happy," Matsunaga says, "with the words mongol, mongolism, and mongoloid, although I agree that they are convenient to use.") The discussion that follows is fairly brief: some agree with Matsunaga, some scientists are dismissive ("an imagined difficulty"), and some try to split the difference, by, for ex-ample, distinguishing between "Mongol" (big *M*, "the racial type") and "mongol" (little *m*, the diagnosis). But beyond the sincere absurdities recorded in the transcript, I wonder what it was really like in the room. What was Matsunaga's tone of voice? What was his body language? Did he pause, gesture, address his comments to a particular colleague? How, in other words, did the unspoken illuminate his speech? It seems to me that Matsunaga's face must have been a silent and eloquent argu-ment. He embodied Down's error.

What to make of the past? How should we commemorate John Langdon Down? Looking back across four decades, or fourteen, it's easy enough to feel superior: *Mongolism* is all but gone, Down's theo-ries long discredited. Do we not live, relatively speaking at least, in an enlightened time? What could be starker than the difference between *Mongolism* and *trisomy 21*, between *idiocy* and *disability*, between a *Mongoloid idiot* and *a person with Down syndrome*? What could be clearer than the difference between Down's blurry racial fancies, and the bright, indisputable contours of chromosomal fact? And yet the actual achievements of Down, not to mention the actual lives of the disabled today, should caution us against complacency. The lesson of the 1966 conference, or of reading John Langdon Down, for that mat-ter, isn't that we're more enlightened than our forebears. It's that they lived in time, and so do we. So we are imperfect and struggling too, making sense of the meanings we inherit—an effort that's difficult, messy, necessary, and still unfinished.

That inheritance is endlessly complex—a fact that came home to me when I finished Ward's biography, and came across a photograph of a family member unmentioned in Lord Brain's centenary invocation. That family member was John Langdon Down: not the scientist, but his grandson. Reginald's son, Stella's brother, Lord Brain's brother-in-law. The youngest child. Though the photograph is a family portrait, it's the boy whose likeness leaps off the page.

John has Down syndrome.

He was born too late to meet his grandfather—his namesake, in every sense—but according to Ward, he was a shock and disappointment to his father. He looks to be about thirteen and is buttoned into a wool suit. He stands behind Stella. He is wearing glasses, and he looks as uncomfortable as any teenage boy who has to hold still for the camera.

Whatever the name applied to the condition—*Mongolian idiocy*, *Down syndrome, trisomy 21*—the people bearing its traces remain a family apart. They inherit *Down* as their second surname. It accompanies the family name, on medical charts, insurance forms, IFSPs. It names a timeless genealogy, a parentless family, in which there are no fathers or mothers, only children who—in Down's view—resemble each other more than they do their own brothers and sisters. In the current debates over naming, in the rejection of something as small as an apostrophe, is the desire to reclaim a child from diagnosis. To say that there are many proper names, and not only one.

Engineering

We were sitting in a Biscuitville in Durham, North Carolina. Ellie's biscuit had butter, and mine had country ham. It was a year after my father had died, and I had left teaching for good, so we were sitting among senior citizens, eating our favorite cheap breakfast, and adjusting to our new life. Ellie was fifteen months old. I got a handful of half-and-halfs from the condiment counter, peeled off the foil lids, and emptied one into my coffee. I lined up the rest like shot glasses in front of Ellie's high chair. She drank out of them one at a time, holding the plastic tubs delicately between finger and thumb.

"Baa," said Ellie.

"Baa," I replied.

"Baa," she said again, and when I followed her eyes to the ceiling-mounted television, I saw Dolly, the cloned sheep.

For a moment, a window opened in the personal, and I noticed something beyond domesticity and grief. I was an unemployed poet and at-home dad in Biscuitville, the youngest retiree in the dining area, and my fifteen-month-old daughter was talking to the image of a clone. It was a good moment to share with Theresa, but when I told her the story, it was more in the spirit of weird news than coming apocalypse. Knowing there was a cloned sheep in a Scottish barn was like knowing about the Central Intelligence Agency daycare, where kids go by first names only: it was a fun fact with a dark side. It was one more example of our modern world.

Years later, I can no longer tell the story in the same way. Our modern world is a little less fun, and issues of genetic control are a little more personal.

We sat and finished our biscuits. I remember the exact, endless luck of a morning with Ellie. It was mixed with the sunlight outside, the smell of indifferent coffee, the salty taste of the ham. Even when being a dad was at its most stressful, icky, or wearisome, I knew my good fortune in my bones: my daughter was a gift beyond anything I could have imagined. At the same time, I spent most of my time thinking that one of us would probably die first, and the other would have to mourn. It was beginning to occur to me that I was maybe more depressed than I had realized. I had always had lousy moods; I had woken up, from time to time, in bleak hotel rooms of the mind. But this was more like a house I had bought. I had moved in, decorated, renovated, rearranged the furniture, and built up substantial equity. I had lived there so long I no longer even felt that depressed.

My father had met Ellie near the end of 1995, when she was two months old and the clock of his prognosis had already run out. When he saw her, he muttered "beauty, beauty," but he could not hold her. Even at ten pounds, she was too heavy for his ribs to bear. I held her just above his chest. A year later, I was writing my way through the memories. During Ellie's naps, I worked on the elegy I had begun while my father was alive. I wrote about missing him and raising Ellie; about cells dividing, some making a tumor, some making a child; about being a writer, the son of an engineer.

And yet I did not link Dolly, the fatherless sheep, the feat of engineering, to any of this. It would take Laura's arrival to show me the relevance of the ewe in the Scottish barn. It is not cloning, exactly, that matters; it is the power cloning implies. That power is fast becoming the context of every family's story.

Three years later, Ellie and I were sitting in a Noah's Bagels in western Oregon. She was drawing a flower, and I was trying to write. I looked at the clock: I had nineteen minutes to go. .

A few months before, we had given in to the obvious fact that Ellie was miserable at her preschool. Set free, she was her sunny self again, but my writing time was gone. So Ellie and I cut a deal. Every morning we would go out for breakfast. When we were done, we would sit together for exactly thirty minutes, during which time I would write poetry and she would draw or color, not disturbing me. I emphasized the "not disturbing" part: except for bathroom breaks, total silence. We'd bring whatever art supplies she needed.

We bought a burgundy-colored three-ring binder and zippered pouches hole-punched to fit inside. We bought markers, pencils, safety scissors, rolls of tape, stickers, fluorescent Post-Its. Ellie sharpened pencils, sorted supplies into pouches. When she was done, she threaded filler paper, gingerly, onto the toothed metal rings of the binder. I snapped the rings shut. Everything was tidy and in its place.

"She gets that from you," I said to Theresa.

And so we began our routine of writing for thirty minutes each day. We'd arrive at Noah's Bagels by midmorning. Ellie lugged her notebook with both arms; my black satchel hung over my shoulder. In it were multiple drafts of the current poem, which had turned out to be about sitting in Noah's Bagels, writing, and glancing over at what Ellie was doing. It was covered with scribbles, emendations, deletions.

We'd lived in Oregon for about two years, and though the Northwest had quickly come to feel like home, being at Noah's reminded me of an older sense of place. I was surrounded by emblematic fragments not of my own childhood, but of my father's: sepia-tinted pictures of old New York, the store's name spelled out in subway tiles. The in-store advertising was a mixture of cornball humor, old-looking newspaper headline fonts, and Yiddish slang, with translations provided. It was nostalgia for outsiders. You could buy and eat the past. You could experiment with new combinations too. You could, in theory, get a Reuben on a blueberry bagel. You could get lox on an "everything" bagel. I tried to imagine what my father would think about *that*.

I had just enough connection left to Judaism to feel proprietary and ironic—but only just enough. I am Jewish by the slimmest of threads, my Japanese mother's conversion. Like New York itself, Judaism is a center I cannot claim, yet both still have some claim on me. Filling Ellie's water cup at the Coke dispenser, glancing at a poster of the Brooklyn Bridge, I experienced a tension, faint but real, between the place I'd come from and the place I'd chosen.

None of this, of course, prevented me from going there each day. The bagels weren't bad, the staff were friendly, and the irritation of faux-Yiddish marketing was outweighed by the wish to be a regular somewhere, in my adopted town. Soon our standard order was ready by the time I got to the register. Once Theresa called me there. I didn't recall anything similar from my own childhood. My parents were solitary and thrifty, and we ate out rarely.

I loved the quiet of working with Ellie. I loved seeing her absorbed in a drawing, tracing a green stem upwards in the middle of a page. But it was my half hour to work, so I turned back to the poem, wondering why I needed to experience things at one remove, filtering my daughter through sentences and lines, in order to see her. I'd glance up now and then, seeing the flower grow in time-lapse. Its stem had two leaves, its petals were yellow. Blades of grass sprouted and clouds appeared. I'd tap a corner of the drawing and say "Nice work," and Ellie would smile, not looking up. If she finished before the half hour was up, she'd say, "Dad," and I'd hold up a finger, write down the last thing I'd thought of, look up, and praise. If she wanted to talk more, I'd say, "Ellie, when the big hand is on the ten." There was a wall clock too, with twelve birds on it. Sometimes we'd look at it together and decide which bird meant we were done. "Dad," she'd say. "It's on the cardinal." It was an article of faith that when the thirty minutes were up, I would put down the mechanical pencil, even in the middle of a sentence.

If you were a professional, my father once told me, you didn't punch a clock. "You work until the job is done," he said. His dedication wove private and public identities, his uncomplaining work ethic and his white-collar job, the one in the city he'd grown up in, then commuted to each day. *Not punching a clock* was a point of pride, because it encapsulated the arc of his life—an upwards arc, an arc of arrival and success, of accomplishments as real as the power plants lighting the suburbs.

Sometimes, on the weekends, I would walk up the creaky stairs to his attic study. He was always glad to see me. He seemed both fascinated with his work and weary of it too. Sometimes he tried to explain what he was working on. The details remain bewildering, the right-angled forest of pipes, the math, but I had the general idea very early on. The radioactive rods heated the water. The water turned to steam, which turned the blades of the turbine, making electricity. Simple.

Once, when I was seven or eight years old, I designed a nuclear car. It was simple, in my head, when I started. By the time I was done, I had a cross between a rat's nest, a Shelby Mustang, and a dirty bomb. There were the uranium rods and then the graphite rods that slid down into the uranium to slow the reaction, so the car could brake for stoplights. I had connected everything with wires and pipes. I had put in bucket seats too. But I had forgotten to shield the passenger compartment from radiation. I remember my dad saying that the lead required would make the car too heavy to run. I remember he told me this truth with affection.

My father spent a couple of years in the army, an experience he advised me to avoid. It is difficult to imagine him there: he was stooped, slope-shouldered, quiet. Recognizing his strengths, the army assigned him to a group of engineers and kept him busy with irrelevant projects. One was a system of springs installed in a truck bed to cushion delicate instruments. In first and second gear, the instruments sat quivering in place as the truck bounced through ruts. In third gear, a mysterious resonance set the springs whanging up and down. Everything broke. On another occasion, he and the engineers were on KP when the vacuum cleaner stopped working. The engineers stooped over the machine, analyzing the failure. Finally the cook—"this big guy," my dad reminisced, "called Cookie"—told the engineers any idiot could see the problem: there was a knot tied in the power cord. They untied the knot, plugged the cord back in, and the vacuum worked.

His career followed the arc of nuclear power. He helped design power plants, and was respected in his office as an engineer's engineer. Eventually he came to think nuclear power was unsafe, that human error would always be impossible to prevent. I don't remember when, exactly, he began to think this, but it may have been after Three Mile Island. He was sent there as a consultant in the aftermath of the disaster. I still remember him showing me a chart on which the pens recording data from the reactor core had run out of ink; on another chart, the ink had overflowed, like a metaphor for meltdown. For critical minutes, there were no data on which to base a decision. I still remember his disgust.

In April of 1995 he had called and said he had a spot on his lung. A few days later he called to say the cancer was terminal. I began looking things up. It was, I thought, what he would do, was not doing, would have done—but *would have done* was wrong. I read about large-cell and small-cell lung cancers, growth rates, needle biopsies, blood tests. I read about the stages of lung cancer. Stages I and II were operable, and IIIa and IIIb were sometimes operable. If your cancer was classified Stage IV, though, there was nothing to do. There was no point in operating on a tumor that had metastasized. So I called my father and asked him what stage he had.

He wasn't sure. They'd said there was nothing to be done. There were sites on both lungs and one on his hip.

"It makes a big difference, though," I said. "If it's IV we can't do anything. If it's IIIb, then maybe we can do something."

I don't remember what he said: A flicker in his voice, then nothing. I rattled off numbers and categories I'd seen, in a source I probably wouldn't have accepted in a student paper. I quoted life expectancies. He listened and didn't say much.

I don't know what I expected: For my father to say, "Thanks, George, that six-to-twelve-month statistic really brightens my day"? For him to seize the possibility of health, the way he'd seized on my one-week-long interest in a math major? I thought I might have found a way out, that we could argue for a clinical trial, bone marrow replacement, *something*. That I could treat cancer as a rhetorical problem, a matter of accurate classification. As I would learn with Laura, much of medicine *is* about rhetoric: logic, categories, negotiated realities. But the central facts were immune to spin. My father was not the hypothetical IIIb, not a candidate for risky but aggressive treatment courses; he was a candidate for the hell of "palliative care," then hospice visits. He had lung cancer, and his first symptom had been a pain in his hip, and there were mets, bad PSA readings, bad white-cell counts. All my statistics were baubles hung on a shadow.

For years afterwards, I thought he was simply in shock at the news, and his empirical common sense had collided with an unimaginable fact. I think now I did not give him enough credit. He was an engineer; the unanticipated was routine. When I remember his stories about knotted power cords, unpredictable resonances, and blooms of spilled ink, I remember the engineer's paradox he lived by: his belief in rational solutions was forever being tested by the misbehavior of the actual world.

Soon after Dolly was unveiled, Ian Wilmut, the project's lead scientist, began receiving calls from the parents of dead children. They wanted to know if their children could be cloned back to life. In the book *After Dolly: The Uses and Misuses of Human Cloning*, which he coauthored with Roger Highfield, Wilmut writes that he began to "dread" these calls. "Cloning," he writes, "does not solve the problem of bereavement." Clones are not duplicates, just as identical twins are not the same: even if Wilmut *could* clone a long-dead child from a lock of hair, the new child would inevitably be different, shaped by culture and cell culture, and would fall short of the expected resurrection.

Although Wilmut opposes reproductive cloning, he has his own pathways between research and loss. In the chapter "Cloning for My Father," Wilmut links his research interest—embryonic stem cells—to the memory of his father's struggle with diabetes. In a description that splices science with longing, Wilmut writes, "Like any son or daughter, I would have done anything to reduce his suffering and make him better. If only there had been a way to halt the underlying disease by replenishing my father's body with his own islet cells, the insulin-producing cells that he lacked." Stem cells, Wilmut explains, have the potential to do so. Later in the chapter, when Wilmut describes how he might save his father, technical details are infused with vivid recollection: "First, I would take a sample of his cells. They could be from the root of a hair or a swab of his cheek . . ."

In that moment, when a future Q-tip swabs a lost cheek, the book moves beyond the General Science category, and becomes something else: a cross between science fiction and elegy. And though Wilmut's life had nothing to do with mine, memory, imagination, and the brain's urge for order and analogy made it all line up: I was reminded of my dad. Part of it was the fact of diabetes, which my father had; but mostly, it was that engineer's *voice*—commonsense, problem-centered, practical—and everything it implied, endless hours in an attic study or in a lab, the dogged care needed to design a power plant, or to clone a sheep.

Beside other projections of our genetic future, Wilmut's seem almost homely. In *Remaking Eden*, for example, the Princeton molecular biologist Lee Silver imagines us engineering our descendants, who in turn engineer their descendants, until after many generations, the human race splits into two species: "Genrich" and "Naturals," the enhanced and the unenhanced, unable to interbreed. In this future, announced with headings like DATELINE WASHINGTON D.C.: MAY 15, 2350, the richest have availed themselves of genes from other animals, giving themselves temperature resistance, the ability to breathe water, and so on. There are sentences like this: "The lung-modified thick-skinned dark green descendants that began their lives on the fourth planet from the sun barely resembled the primitive *Naturals* still roaming the planet Earth." On the one hand, Silver clearly sees dystopic elements to a future in which Genrich and Naturals no longer breed. On the other hand, he seems to think that it could be really, really cool.

In Silver's projection, this future begins with parents only wanting the best for their children. Mere cloning will seem primitive: we will be able to tinker with the human genome itself, not only to prevent disease, but to select genes for desired traits. In time, according to Silver, scientists will be able to forge artificial chromosomes containing "gene-packs" for traits deemed positive, like mathematical ability. Parents will be able to shop for these "gene-packs" and insert them into embryos. Having an extra chromosome will signify something different than it does now.

I wonder about Down syndrome, in a future of increasing power over the genome. We live in a world where Down syndrome is described both as an element of a diverse humanity and as a defect to be eliminated. Our medicine embodies this doubleness—we use open-heart surgery to save infants with Down syndrome, and an array of tests to keep from having these infants in the first place—and whatever we think about Down syndrome in the future, our medicine will embody that too.

I don't think Down syndrome will disappear: for that to happen, screening would have to become universal. Nor is it likely to be the object of "enhancement": if a prospective parent is choosing between, say, musical ability and athletic ability, then Down syndrome as an option will simply be off the table. But it may become rare. People with Down syndrome have had a long, uncertain journey from invisibility, to racialized diagnosis, to the beginnings of citizenship, but there is no guarantee their progress will continue. Whether it does, and whether our emerging technologies help them in their journey, depends largely on how they are seen—and, in particular, how public scientists like Lee Silver and Ian Wilmut, who not only develop the technologies but shape opinion about policy, see them.

After Dolly and *Remaking Eden* are very different books, but in one way they are alike: Down syndrome, despite all that has been learned, told, and amply witnessed, remains an abstraction. It is presented as a technical problem, as an example of genetic abnormality, and as an example of the sort of thing reproductive technology can save us from. But the people with Down syndrome don't rate a story; they are not given the human reality that is granted to the author, to other scientists, to hypothetical characters facing reproductive decisions, and even to green-skinned, lung-modified descendants leaving an overcrowded planet.

If our technologies are to benefit people with Down syndrome, then their lives need to become more real to us. Science can illuminate one part of that reality, and technology can affect it. But only story can convey it.

January 2004

Every family has one toy it cannot get rid of. Ours is the Fisher-Price Talking Smart Street.

It was given to us by Theresa's sister Susie, who passed it on with wicked glee, when Ellie was about one: I'd made fun of it so often, as my nephew Randy played with it, that she thought I should have it. Over the years I have tried to give it to friends with younger children. The children lug it away wide-eyed, as their parents glare back darkly from the door. Like a psychopathic orphan, the toy always comes back.

It has a kind of upright facade, like a Hollywood stage set, about a foot high and a foot and a half wide. Though its organizing principle is a street, it is more like a minimall, with a music store (a set of keys in a major scale), a post office (a slot for a plastic letter), a bank, and a town clock, which reports the time when you move its hands. When it talks, it does so in the stereotypical voice of a nerdy adult male: nasal, nonthreatening, enthusiastic, a little high-pitched. There is no volume control. I mimic the voice, for Ellie's benefit; she mimics the mimicry. I play its chromatic melody on the piano, a tinny fanfare evocative of carousels, ice-cream trucks, and the fun of learning. Its score is seared deep into my cortex. When I am on my deathbed, my lungs deflating for the last time in a ring of friends, family, and hospice personnel, I expect to hear the electronic chime of the Smart Street song, and a nasal voice welcoming me to the afterlife.

Parents who have been suckered out of hundreds of dollars by the promise of "interactivity" will know what I mean when I say that the Talking Smart Street is more of a talker than a listener, and that if patience is a part of learning, the Talking Smart Street is an enemy of education. It is a needy, difficult companion. It says, "Welcome to Smart Street! Turn the dial!" It says, "Let's visit the music store!" It says, "Find *A*! Let's visit the clock!" It is inflexible in its suggestions, and it dislikes being ignored. Laura stabs at buttons, and it says, "Sorry! Try again," or "That's . . . *L*! Find . . . *A*!" Eerie, inhuman gaps in the nerd's speech, the algorithms not quite ironed out, as if Laura were dialing up flight arrival information: automation claiming agency, the weirdness of a machine that says "I." What can it mean when the Talking Smart Street says "Good job"? What satisfaction, from recorded praise?

It does not educate; it distracts. And though I hate the thing in principle, I keep it around, because it will distract Laura, for a few minutes anyway. Too tired to live up to my invective, I say, "Here, play with this"; and like every parent who swears his child won't be polluted by TV, by video games, by meat, I bridge the gap with irony. I say, "Hey, Ellie, I need to get dinner together. Whyn't you guys play with Smart Street." And they do. I chop onions, move the laundry through, or, guiltily, hurriedly, check e-mail, addicted to distractions of my own.

Lately, like HAL singing "A Bicycle Built for Two," the Talking Smart Street has begun to go off the rails. It may be suffering from a stress disorder. It says, "Find. . . zero . . . o'clock!" It confuses the music store with the pet store. It says, "Find . . . L!"

Ellie, sitting with Laura on the ugly, unreplaced carpet of the living room, helps Laura find L. She presses Laura's finger to L.

It says, "Sorry! Find . . . L!"

Ellie has a strict and unfailing sense of justice. She howls from the living room: "Dad, it asked for L and I pressed L and it said I was WRONG!"

"It's okay, honey," I say. "The batteries are running down."

All parents are futurists, and every toy is an idea of the future: we want our children to be talking and smart, because we believe this will help them be happy. These are the kind of wishes that seem obvious and uncomplicated, until a child with Down syndrome comes along.

Laura has a way of altering my vision, in ways both big and small. After Laura, Dolly meant something different. But then, so did the Talking Smart Street. Taking care of my daughters, reading Ian Wilmut and Lee Silver, I saw our household toys in a different way. The Talking Smart Street. The geometrical wood puzzle, with its label that blares MAKES YOUR CHILD SMARTER! The black-and-white mobile. We didn't think these things would make Ellie smarter, any more than we believed the Talking Smart Street would make Laura talk. Nor did we see anything wrong with teaching Laura to talk, whether through mobile, book, or electronic LeapPad. But at the same time, the toys seemed evidence of a ravenous, not always pretty desire to improve our children. The logic is not just that Talking + Smart = Happy. It's that you can *buy* your way to Talking and Smart. How else to explain the plethora of choices in the toystore? How else to explain the brand names: Bright Baby, Baby Einstein, Smart Baby? And what, exactly, drives the purchasing decision? At what point does the desire for Smart shade into the fear of Not-Smart—or can those impulses be separated at all?

To be Laura's dad is to be orphaned from the great certainties. In the bookstore I walk past racks of books *For Dummies* and *Idiot's Guides*. In the movie theater I once sat silent, watching *Borat*, the crowd convulsed around me at retard jokes—and we say *convulsed* with laughter, because the jokes, for all their wit, for all the intelligence that sharpens a point, drives it home, and twists, depend on something subrational, instinctive, animalistic. On the softball field, a frat boy at shortstop: "Dude, I felt like such a retard, making that error." Once, in the coffee shop in the basement of the Valley Library, I heard a woman say to a table of friends, "What do you have, a *trisomy* or something?" The table broke up in laughter. Our jokes, as more than one writer has pointed out, are all diagnoses—*idiot, moron, retard, trisomy.*

That equation of intellect with human value is difficult to see, and likely impossible to transcend. But it is reflected in our jokes, our toys, and our movies, and if we choose to engineer future human beings, it will be reflected in their bodies. Our technology lends force to what we believe.

The appeal of the Talking Smart Street is no different than the appeal of Silver's imagined gene-packs. The only difference is that the gene-packs, in theory at least, will work better. Instead of setting an irritating toy in front of your tot, you'll program the pre-tot embryo. Instead of nurture, you'll change nature. For advocates of this approach, genetic engineering is simpler and more effective. But for critics, the bright future has a dark side. Bill McKibben, the author of *Enough: Staying Human in an Engineered Age*, points out that, as with anabolic steroids in baseball players, the drive to alter biology diminishes the meaning of the accomplishment. It is the ultimate expression of control over a child, and the antithesis of accepting that child for herself. And to a degree unimaginable for today's marketers, it makes the child herself a consumer product.

Like all products, McKibben points out, that child's software will become obsolete: she'll be better than her nonengineered peers, but worse than the next generation. The problem is, she'll be stuck with her out-of-date software. The irony is that in a continual "arms race" for improvement, as McKibben calls it, the improved are destined to be inferior. Silver's oddly dystopic vision—in which the "GenRich" and "Naturals" are unable to interbreed—is the logical endpoint of this arms race.

Reading *Remaking Eden*, I was struck by one hypothetical enhancement: the ability to see beyond the visible spectrum, and "into the ultraviolet range." It occurred to me that I'd been seeing in ultraviolet since Laura was born. In the bookstore, the toystore, the coffee shop, the movie theater, the world fluoresced, as if a black light were shining everywhere. That light cast itself across memory too, highlighting old pictures in a new way: my dad in the attic with a diagram of wires and pipes. Ellie, in a restaurant in North Carolina, saying "baa" to the TV image of a clone.

In that light, even the Talking Smart Street looks a little strange. It is, like Silver's imaginary gene-packs, a consumer product that appeals to an ordinary parental wish, one we share: to help our children do a little better. The difference, apart from effectiveness, is mainly in the engineering.

It was the spring of 2000, the new millennium, and despite the miscellaneous predictions of apocalypse, our life looked much the same. Ellie and I were still writing together. I finished the poem, and in April, we found Ellie a new preschool. Like most of the parents I know, I love my children very much, and I do best with a few hours of childcare each day. Ellie, I think, was a little relieved.

But we kept to our daily writing schedule, because—well, it worked for me. I started a second poem called "Codes." It was autobiographical. It had three principal characters: my mom, Ellie, and me. It included my mother's gnomic statements about writing and life and pain; it included my childhood memories of hearing her typewriter through the closed study door. As I wrote, Ellie copied me across the table, making long, looping scribbles. In the poem, I equated that scribble with the long signatures of DNA: beneath the script of nurture that linked my mom, Ellie, and me, beneath Japanese and English, DNA was a common language, the deep script we shared. One long argument, beneath all the arguments. The poem was filled with gene-words, like *transcription* and *recombination*. It's obvious now that my obsession with genes and generations was triggered not only by Ellie but by her nameless sibling, whose kicks Theresa was then beginning to feel. This one was different, Theresa said. It wanted to use her bladder as a trampoline.

I finished the poem in the fall. Then I began renovating the upstairs bathroom.

When Laura arrived, the poem seemed instantly absurd—one more irony in the cornucopia of irony my life had become. All my meditations had assumed a normal child. I had thought of the molecule as a script of connection, of likeness descending the generations. But the billions of letters we had counted on to spell out happiness, as they had with Ellie, now seemed a giant anagram of misery and regret.

Laura was born a few days after the "Draft of the Human Genome" was published: the detailed transcription, letter by letter, of every human chromosome. It is, in a way, the ultimate personal essay—one normal person, one typical man, standing for all. It is a necessary prelude to genetic engineering: to change a gene, you have to know what and where it is. And it is a feat of engineering in its own right, a massive, computer-driven project, wherein samples of pure DNA were "shotgunned"—broken into short fragments, then read, reread, and assembled by computer. It seemed my life had been shotgunned too, broken into uncountable pieces that would have to be reassembled into a legible picture of the whole. I soon learned I was wrong, that my life had not been shattered. But by then I was writing a book. I was awash in fragments of my own.

By the spring of 2004, Laura was three years old, and I'd been working on a book about her for nearly as long. Though I had given up poetry for prose, I was still writing about genes and generations, just as I had while sitting with Ellie beneath the pictures of old New York. But after Laura, I couldn't write about genes in the same way. I couldn't use words like *transcription* and *recombination* for purely literary value, and I couldn't just sing about the links between the generations, because we lived in a world that held Dolly the sheep. If the power implied by Dolly's existence is likely to increase and to be used, then our stories matter, because we are deciding who gets to have a story in the first place. We are deciding who counts, and what kind of story is worthwhile.

How, then, to tell Laura's story? How to explain the way my vision had changed? Because by then, Laura had long been one of us, a fully vested member of our family, and the happiness she brought us was real, without dilution or asterisk. She was a part of our story. Her trisomy had complicated that story, from heart surgery to speech therapy. But her genetic beginnings—on paper, far less promising than Ellie's—had resulted in no less happiness. The genome is the beginning of the story, not the end.

In time, I came to see our situation this way: Laura has a double inheritance. Like Ellie, Laura inherits the extraordinary luck of an American middle-class life: she's loved, insured, and free. But unlike Ellie, she was born with a recognizable genetic disorder. As a result, she also inherits a history of misunderstanding—and our anxieties about what our chromosomes have to do with who we are.

Theresa said once that Laura has Laura syndrome, that I have George syndrome, that Ellie has Ellie syndrome: we all have our risk factors. The difference, with Laura, is that her risk factors are *known*.

Because chromosomes are easy to see under the microscope, because people with Down syndrome have a distinctive appearance, and because Down syndrome has been extensively studied, we could have that knowledge for one child and not another. But for parents in the near future, and perhaps for all of us, that distinction may be coming to an end.

There may never be a human clone, or a green-skinned Martian colonist, or even a child engineered for musical ability. But the era of personalized genomic medicine, long predicted, is all but here. In the wake of the Human Genome Project, it is now possible to "sequence," letter by letter, a full set of human chromosomes. A few people have already had this done, and though having a full personal reading of the Book of Life is still too expensive for you and me, it will soon be commonplace: as the price of a finished sequence comes down, we will each come to possess the Book we already own. We will carry it to the doctor's office—on a compact disk, on an iPod—and we will live our lives by the Book, adjusting our medical choices to its predictions. We will have numbers for everything, for heart disease, lung cancer, diabetes, depression, Alzheimer's, Parkinson's, obesity. We may, in some cases, have better medical interventions to choose from. But even when we have no cure, we will still have the numbers.

In other words, we will all know our syndromes. In this way, at least, Laura—born days after the publication, in *Nature* and *Science*, of the draft of who we are—is typical of us all. Her inheritance is ours.

March 2004

I hear the car pull in and the doors open and shut. Then Ellie runs up the walk and the door slams behind her.

"Where's Mom and Laura?" I ask.

"They're in the car. Laura's really crabby, she keeps saying 'd'bin, d'bin,' and we don't know what it means."

Ellie goes into her art room and shuts the door. I hear Laura's wailing approaching the front door, like a distant train. Then the door opens, and Theresa has Laura under her left arm. Laura is weeping. "D'bin," she says, "d'bin." Theresa sighs.

"D'pen" is "Penny." "D'bee" is "book." "D'feen" is "swing." We don't know "d'bin."

"What's 'd'bin,' Laura?" I ask.

"D'bin," she says, tears in her eyes. "D'bin, d'bin."

"Hey Laura," I say. "Do you want to watch TV? And eat chips?"

"Da!" she says, enthusiastically. "Da! D'tthep!" And she toddle-sprints towards the back room where the TV is. In fifteen seconds I will hear *DAT!* She will want to know where the chips are.

Three days later, I'm downtown with Ellie and Laura, killing the afternoon: fly shop, coffee shop, practice crossing streets safely, the usual. Then Laura points at the bookstore, and says: "D'bin!"

"Hey El," I say, "look at that. She meant 'the Book Bin.'"

The sound Ellie makes is difficult to describe.

After Ellie, what did we expect from a second child? Laura's diagnosis taught us that comparison, though inevitable, was pointless. We were starting over, whether we liked it or not. Down syndrome only drove the point home.

When Laura arrived, we did not know who she was. And then, when the test came back, it seemed the scales had fallen from our eyes. We had been living an illusion of normalcy, and now we knew the truth. In retrospect, I think we had only entered into a deeper ignorance. We still did not know who Laura was; and then, in shock, we didn't know what we didn't know. In this way, too, Laura is more like Ellie than unlike: when Ellie was born, she was a total mystery. With Laura, the ordinary mysteries were slower to arrive.

But to compare them is false, because we love them equally—if "equally" can mean anything, where numerical values are irrelevant—and because they didn't take turns. First there was Ellie; then there was

Ellie-and-Laura. We had one child, then two; and it's the fact of two, more than the differences between them, that shapes my days.

When we were waiting for Laura to come along, I was mainly worried about what it was like to have two kids, instead of one. Then, for a while, that question vanished, and I was thinking about Down syndrome. And then Down syndrome became ordinary—or as ordinary as it could be, in a world where it is vanishing, feared, welcomed, and strange—and what everyone had told me turned out to be true after all. *The second child changes everything.*

Increments and Fates

When we were eighteen years old and our intensely repressed academic courtship had barely begun, Theresa said something about molecules: that tiny quantities of them could make a difference in whether you knew what day it was, or whether you remembered your name. We were talking all the time then, each figuring out how to get the other one to stick around longer, and most of what we said has settled into the thin, compacted layers of The Days When We First Met; but what Theresa said about molecules has stayed with me, like a prophecy that actually panned out.

Carbon-dated fragments—*Watson dormitory, University of Virginia, wire-rimmed glasses*—put the conversation in early 1983. I remember the molecule idea struck me as kind of weird. I still owned my battered pink copy of *Zen and the Art of Motorcycle Maintenance*, and I had also read *Ulysses*, though I had not understood it. I was going to be a writer. I had confidently decided that science was irrelevant to me.

But I liked being with Theresa. I had been unaccountably unhappy for a long time, and I had temporarily solved the problem by retreating to the windowless bunker of my moods. In Theresa I had met someone worth coming out for. By extension, the world was worth coming out for too.

There were, of course, adjustments. It still amazes me that we survived the apple. We had gone apple-picking that fall, when it was obvious to everyone but us that we would soon be dating. I left one of the apples on my windowsill, then forgot about it. One day I drew back the curtain and noticed it was discolored and sagging. I decided to track its progress. Theresa's pleas to throw it out rose gradually in pitch, but I refused. Soon it dried and began to shrivel. At the end of the year, it was much lighter.

Sometimes, after we began dating, I would leave her apartment beneath a personal, Linus-sized black cloud, my face set in what I knew was an unhelpful, impassive mask. Behind me, she was kicking the wall. I didn't know. I herded my little demons to the bus. I went to the library, I went to class, I went off to work on a poem. I would call later and say I was sorry. She would say it was only receptors. I could almost hear her almost smiling. When I read between the lines of her voice, I heard her thinking that the molecules mattered, that I probably could not help sinking into my moods, but that a molecular jerk is no less a jerk. She had, somehow, kindness and science in balance. She was able to live with contradiction. These are useful qualities, if you happen to have a daughter with Down syndrome.

After we graduated, we set off on our road trip. I'd visited Japan, but had never been west of Buffalo. Rooted in New York, settled and solitary, my parents had never seen much reason to go inland, and perched warily on the continent's edge. But Theresa's parents were both born in Pittsburgh, and her roots in the country are deeper than mine. In Kentucky we visited her mother's cousins, Ed and Becky. They were in their sixties; Ed had retired from the navy years before, and they were living beside a reservoir. Ed had a big boat. I asked about the fishing, and he said it was good. I felt at home with them, as I do, less often, with people my own age: though the terms of my relationship with Theresa were vague, and though I was as out of place in rural Kentucky as E.T., I seemed to impress them as a nice young man. In the morning we were awakened at seven for breakfast on good china (scrambled eggs, country ham, orange juice). Then we said good-byes, headed blearily west towards I-40, and the trip was our own.

For a few days we bore an uncertain silence across the baking

Midwest. After a postapocalyptic campground in Oklahoma—an oily sheen to the river, the showers working fine but the sites abandoned—the mood began to lighten, and then we arrived in the fenced-off spaces of the West. I was born in the nervous center of the world, I was raised in the dendritic jumble of its suburbs, and I could not comprehend the raw scale of New Mexico. We flew across the land, but crawled across the map. The mountains kept their distance, like a mirage.

It didn't matter how fast we went. We got lost in long twisting conversations on straight roads and bore a comfortable quiet up twisting canyons. We listened to Elvis Costello and the B-52s on the boom box until the batteries faded—the plain brown Corolla, a sensible shoe of a car if there ever was one, had only an AM radio. We bought new batteries. We took pictures on a camera with film. We kept a ledger, so we could settle up at the end of the trip: I was moving to Ithaca, Theresa to Philadelphia, and though it was clear that if we could survive weeks together we could survive them apart, the autumn was an open question.

I feel old recounting it, nostalgic for the days of pay phones and floppy disks, when hard drives were measured in kilobytes and gas cost less than a dollar a gallon, when it was possible to drive cross-country without thinking about atmospheric warming, and the flags were not ordinarily at half-mast. We did not see a single Starbucks, not even one.

After Arches National Park, Theresa announced that she was tired of red rocks, and we began heading towards San Francisco. We crossed the Mojave Desert with a mask and snorkel perched on top of our luggage: for the whole trip I had been hoping to find clear water somewhere, so I could swim around in it and look at fish. I did not use it until we arrived in British Columbia. Theresa still mentions the snorkel, though mostly with affection.

If we went through Corvallis then, I don't remember it. Oregon was the big square thing between San Francisco and Seattle; I remember driving along the coast at sunset, and a pancake house on I-5 with tractor-trailers in the parking lot. I remember it was raining.

March 2005

It's been another dry, eerily mild winter, like the year Laura was born. The reservoirs draw down; vast wildfires are predicted for the summer. The daffodils come up three weeks early. Laura and I sit on the sidewalk, waiting for the bus to take her to Dixie School, where she receives special education services in a classroom setting. She's four years old now, old enough to ride the school bus on her own.

I write a T in white chalk on the concrete. I say, "Laura, can you trace *T*?"

"Per-puh," she says, and I hand her the purple chalk. She traces a ragged *T*, like a shadow cast by mine. I am so happy, saying, "Yay Laura, yes!" She pumps her fist and says, "Ess!"

She's speaking more clearly now. In the fall, she had tubes placed in her ears to correct a moderate hearing loss; her tonsils and adenoids came out too. Soon afterwards, her articulation began to improve. We noticed it particularly in the vowels: long *a*, short *a*, *o* and *oo*. Debbie McPheeters, then Laura's speech-language pathologist, speculated that the reason she'd always done better with consonants—*p*, *b*, *m*—was that she'd been lip-reading. You can't *see* the difference between long and short *a*.

But Laura still found speech difficult. Her solution was to use the same word for multiple meanings—*bop*, for instance, could mean *pizza*, *stop*, or *potty*—and clarify the different meanings with her hands. Saying *bop* while signing *eat* meant *pizza*; while doing a karate chop against the palm, *stop*; while patting her rear, the elusive but slowly improving *potty*. At some point it struck me that Laura was signing while she spoke, exactly the way Pat Hill had shown us how to do years ago, when we hardly knew what Down syndrome was.

I hear the familiar diesel engine, and the yellow bus trundles around the corner and pulls up in front of the house. I say hi to the driver, lift Laura into her seat, buckle her in, kiss her, and tell her to be good. As the bus pulls away, she is waving to me from the window.

Four mornings a week, Laura attends a second preschool—the Oregon State University Child Development Center, known also as Bates Hall. Laura is the only child with Down syndrome there. At Bates, Laura receives no services, but she is learning how to be with other children, and they are learning how to be with her.

One morning I arrive early for pickup. I go inside, sit down in the Observation Room, and unfold my laptop. Over the glow of that day's searches, I watch Laura through a wall of one-way glass. It's time for Large Group, and the class is singing "The Wheels on the Bus," Laura's favorite song. Laura sits on her carpet square and rotates her fists one over the other, backup-singer style, for "Round and Round," claps her hands together for "Open and Shut," swings a thumb up over her shoulder for "Move on Back." She loves Large Group. At first she needed someone to sit behind her, but she knows the routine now.

That Laura is part of the group, that she sits cooperatively on her carpet square, is an achievement. Shahrnaz Badiee, the dark-haired, brisk, affectionate head teacher, has made it her business to teach Laura how things work, to hold her—insofar as possible—to the same standards as other children, and to help the other children understand her. Shahrnaz is one of the many adults without whom *inclusion* would be a meaningless word. To include a child like Laura is not necessarily difficult, but it does take commitment.

After Large Group comes Small Group. Laura is not cooperating. She is staging her sit-down strike, refusing to go to the Library Area. Laura says *anh*, reaches for the sky, denying the handhold of her armpits. I start to get up, to go inside and intervene, then think better of it. Shahrnaz comes over, talks gently to Laura, then firmly lugs her to Small Group. The Library Area is directly opposite my chair. Laura makes faces at herself in the mirror, gesturing, in one of her hermetic stories. It looks as if she's talking to me.

I fold up the laptop and unplug it and put it away, and then I sling its weight over my shoulder. I leave the ambery twilight of Observation; the classroom is bright and loud. Shahrnaz says, "Look Laura, look who's here!" And Laura barrels across the room towards me, in the way Ellie used to, when *she* went to Bates Hall. At nine, Ellie is far too old for public hugs. Laura, however, is still incapable of reserve. She throws her arms around me, the best part of the day. Then I take her to the potty, and we go outside to the tire swing.

I have acquired minor fame at the Bates Hall playground, where, for those kids who sit on the swing with Laura, I do the full-on clown routine. I pretend to get knocked down by the swing, then do somersaults and come up covered with bark chips. I pretend to take naps until the kids wake me up with their screaming. I pretend to misplace the children. "Lara, Olivia, Laura," I say, "where are you?" Their orbit decays. I search for them in my wallet and under the bark chips. When the screaming gets too loud—"WE'RE RIGHT HERE," with Laura echoing, "ERE"—I discover them, then ask why they didn't say something earlier.

It is the way I play with children when I am not depressed, but it is also a calculated game of inclusion. Since it is about momentum and silliness and screaming, and not, say, numeracy, Laura's deficits become temporarily irrelevant. Besides, I'm happy to embarrass myself for her sake. If the kids associate Laura with Fun, Laughter, and Incompetent Clown Dad, that's fine by me. It beats the hell out of Weird-Looking Kid Who Can't Talk.

I say, "Okay, guys, five more minutes!" We have to get home in time for the bus. The kids protest. I give them a last push and they scream with happiness. Laura is screaming too, saying, "ZOOM! ZOOM!" The other kids think Laura is saying *zoom* because they're going fast, so they say it too. But Laura is saying *zoom* because *zoom* is how Laura says *more*. It was Theresa who figured out the etymology. In daily life, we don't say "more"; we say "some more," as in, "Do you want some more O's and milk?" Laura chose, for whatever reason, to contract the phrase to *some*, which she pronounces *zoom*. We say, "Laura, look at me. MORE." "ZOOM," she says. She likes it. We know what it means. She owns *zoom*. In general, it is difficult to sway her, once her mind is made up—though what looks like stubbornness may only be a difficulty in changing course.

We say *more*, and it comes back *zoom*; we say *TV*, and it comes back *Bobo*. The etymology was, again, complex and personal. *Bobo* was Laura's best pronunciation of *Elmo*, which stood, in general, for TV. Therefore: *Bobo* = TV. *Bobo* could also refer specifically to Elmo, in the way that *bread* can denote either bread or food in general. Give us this day our daily Bobo. We spent a lot of time clarifying which Bobo Laura meant, how much Bobo she could have, and whether she could have chips along with Bobo. Sometimes, to make her case that Bobo should be allowed right now, and in unlimited quantities, Laura would drag out the old invented sign for TV, flicking her fingers beneath her chin. We said no, signing for emphasis. Or we caved and agreed. We consented, in every way, to her terms.

Since the beginning, she has been teaching us. She translates our messages; we retranslate the translation. We say *zoom* and *Bobo*. We say *oop* instead of *oops*: Laura, for reasons of her own, deleted the trailing "s." Others learned her language too. Lara, a tire swing regular who had become something that once seemed as improbable as a unicorn—a friend—had begun saying "Da" around the house. When her father asked what it meant, she told him, "That's how you say *yes* in Laura."

But there's more than one way to say *yes* in Laura. Sometimes she nods once, an imperial inclination of the head. Sometimes she says *yes* uncertainly, as a conversational placeholder; sometimes, the way a tourist says *yes*, meaning "I don't totally understand, I missed that, but I still want to be a part of things here." Sometimes—when she does understand, and is understood—her *yes*, her *da*, is triumphant, delighted: "Daaaaayy!"

She insists *U* is *Q*. She says *eight* is *ett*. If I switch routes while driving home, she screams her version of *other way*: "athay! ATHAY!" She contracts sentences to words and words to fragments. We understand some, try to decipher the rest. We play twenty questions, following winding, Socratic paths towards simple facts: the skinned knee, what she did at school. Still, we have clarities, precisions, we did not dream of a year ago. Her speech is a landscape before dawn: indistinct shapes, a darkness textured by the eye. It brightens towards an imagined, articulate noon. It was true of Ellie once, at the same developmental, if not calendar, age. *Bah* for *bye*, *lellow* for *yellow*: everything we are charmed by, and want to correct.

Down syndrome did not transform our lives, so much as expose its basic terms. That we struggle to understand each other sometimes, that the nonverbal cues are often louder and clearer than the spoken ones, seems only a special case of what is commonly true.

April 2005

Another global warming sunny day. We sit, doodle, wait for the bus. I ask Laura which animal she wants me to draw.

"B-guh."

I say, "Look at me." I hold up two fingers before her, a hypnotist. I tap my lips, pronounce /b/. "B-b-bug." She says, "K-k-k-buzza." "No, Laura," I say, "B-b-bug." She says, "B-buz-buzza." I'm happy with that. I say, "Good try! Good job! High five!" I draw the bug, which is basically a potato with two eyes, a mouth, and six legs like commas. The deluxe bug has antennae. I can also draw dogs, horses, sharks, elephants, and flowers. It is a limited repertoire, but good enough for grocery store checkout lines, airport boarding areas, and waiting for the bus. Over the week, the pictograms accumulate and fade on the sidewalk, as though centuries were passing in a cave.

"Dan!" says Laura.

"Dad," I say. "Say Dad."

"Dat!" she says.

"What, Laura?"

"Da peen!"

The plane! The plane, boss, the plane! We are playing the home version of *Fantasy Island*. She is Hervé Villechaize, and I am Ricardo Montalban. The wealthy visitors are arriving to live out their dreams, the ones they always knew would bring them happiness, but did not dare to hope for: I want to raise a child with Down syndrome!

It is just an airplane. I hadn't noticed it, but I know the story that is coming, the story she always tells. She points. "Da ky," she says. The sky. Next, I know, she will say what she always says.

"Mum mum da peen."

"That's right," I say. "Mum mum rode on the plane."

"La la da peen."

"Yup. Ellie rode on the plane."

"Dat da peen."

"Dad rode on the plane too."

She tells stories for the same reason we do: because something interesting happened, because it matters to her for some reason she cannot account for, and because telling the story—the act of it, and the act of being heard—means that she belongs. Once, when we were all sitting at dinner, she interrupted the laughter over a joke she did not understand:

"Dat!"

"What, Laura."

"Eh heh heh heh."

Eh heh heh heh is Laura's not-real laugh, the one she makes to explain that she gets the concept of laughing, that things can be funny, and that she is capable of joining in with us, though she doesn't quite get the joke this time.

We all cracked up, because it was cute, and Laura said, "Mam!"

"What, Laura."

"Eh heh heh heh heh."

I draw pictures of us on the sidewalk, and label them MOM, DAD, ELLIE, LAURA. Everyone is a stick figure, except for Laura. She stands beside us on stout body and stubby legs, the only solid thing in a planar world.

To *advocate*, in special-needs jargon, is to speak up on a child's behalf. There are many possible advocates, and many forms of advocacy, but to me the term covers IEP meetings, a brief chat with a teacher after school, a few minutes pushing the tire swing, taking Laura out with me everywhere, writing a book. To advocate is to be teacher, ambassador, interpreter, storyteller. It is everything I do to help others imagine Laura.

At Bates Hall, at the beginning of every term, Shahrnaz and I would sit down with the new student teachers, and I would advocate for Laura. I covered Down syndrome (what it is, Laura's health status, common misconceptions), language (Laura's signs and fragmentary words), potty (coming along), food (fries, chips, rice, nuggets, good luck with everything else), behavior (occasionally stubborn, loves to learn, wants to belong). I talked about social challenges: that when other children pointed out that she was different, or that she couldn't do something, the best approach was to shift the paradigm. To have Laura show some of her signs, for example. The idea was to redefine Laura as capable in some way, thus finding common ground. I also asked the student teachers to model treating Laura as ordinary. To speak to her in the same voice they used for the other children, for example, and not in the high, squeaky voice used for babies.

I have a terrible memory for both faces and names, so most of the student teachers have long since blurred into a vague parade of Meghans, Ashleys, and Caitlins. But Laura, I know, left a more durable imprint. Often, at the end of the term, at least one student was in tears, telling me how much Laura had taught her. Time and again, I have seen the adults in Laura's life—the babysitters, volunteers, student teachers, friends, physical therapists, early intervention coordinators—try to articulate what Laura meant to them. Since the beginning of her life, she has left people at a loss for words.

Laura does not merely charm people; she dawns on them. In her particularity, she both opposes and exposes the composite portrait— half li'l angel, half tragedy—that reigns in the public mind. She tends to surprise people, though usually it is after they think they know her. Teachers, friends, babysitters inevitably witness Darth Laura for the first time (polite version: "she's feisty," or "she does have a temper"), or she does something—solves a puzzle, says a word they understand, or shows she understands them—which bears witness to a human intelligence, complex, different, and real.

I have come to see that Laura is her own best advocate. If the preconceptions are at least set aside, if her diagnosis can be seen accurately and she can be seen as distinct from her diagnosis, then she can handle it from there.

One day that summer, Theresa came home after a lousy day at work and decided she could no longer live with the ochre shag carpet I had meant to replace for six years. This sparked what I think she might refer to as a "signaling cascade." It was as if there were neurons responsible purely for being annoyed about the carpet, and those fired or upregulated or whatever it is they do, and in doing so they upregulated the pantry neurons, the downstairs bathroom neurons, the deck neurons, the roof moss neurons, and the still-not-quite-finished-since-before-Laura's-birth upstairs bathroom neurons, and together they produced the conviction in my wife that it was time to call someone to finish the house. Then we would either like it and continue to live there, or the house would be ready to sell, and we would move. Where we would move to was an open question, but Ellie was ten. She could use her own room anyway.

In the summer of 2005, we did everything I'd meant to do, when we first moved in. We fixed up the downstairs bathroom, replaced single-pane windows, bolted handrails beside the stairs. We fixed the deck, which had buckled over the winter: in the years we'd lived there, the tree had grown to fill the hole cut for its passage. When I say "we," I say it in the way most people say it: we paid a licensed contractor to do it. I pitched in, putting the book aside. I tiled the kitchen and pantry, built new pantry cabinets and doors. It felt good to be working again, but it was just work. In the spring we had the house painted yellow and red. Even before we put the house on the market, it looked like someone else's. It sold in two days. We bought a ranch house where Ellie would have her own room and where, as Theresa said, everything was *done*.

In the month before closing, we put back the echoes. We filled three Dumpsters with accumulated trash, with dead appliances and Happy Meal toys and trash left by the owners before us. I emptied the shed, setting eight years of renovation's leftovers by the curb, plywood scraps and buckets of joint compound, coiled wire and lengths of pipe and half-gallons of paint. They were scavenged immediately. I am a packrat by nature, but I was getting in the spirit of things. I even set out the broken electric mandolin, which had begun to disintegrate in storage. On my way home with a new package of file boxes, I saw a stranger with an enormous handlebar mustache, bicycling away from my house, holding up the mandolin in triumph.

On the day we handed the keys over, the house smelled like Windex. The carpets were vacuumed, the cobwebs broomed out, the sills dusted, the new tile floors mopped, the windows spotless. Ellie walked through the house with the digital camera, documenting. She photographed everything I'd built in place, as if we would always live there. On the computer, the photos look like candidates for a magazine spread: *Amateur Renovation, Procrastinating Author.*

For days afterwards, the house continued to change. A new fence went up. The rhododendrons were torn out. So were the stumps in the front yard, where an arborist we knew had taken down two scraggly pines, chainsawed the stumps into chairs, then traced *E* and *L* on the chairs with the chainsaw's tip. We weren't sad about these things: it was their house now. The only one to disagree was Laura. "Om," she said, as we drove by, and we said, "No, Laura! That's our old *house!* We're going *home!*" For weeks she refused to concede the point. She was utterly clear: the new place was "ahse," just a house. The old place was "om."

Science is Theresa's country, not mine. For years I have felt like a tourist, awash in the strangeness of its surfaces. After I moved to Philadelphia, when Theresa was still finishing her PhD, science was the fluorescent quiet in a lab after midnight, as we went in to feed Theresa's cells. It was dry ice, calculators, labeled flasks sealed with foil. It was a column of numbers, in Theresa's handwriting, on the tea-stained page of a lab notebook. In the years since, as Theresa became a postdoc, then a professor, it became the jargon of her grants, *phospholipase, monomer, cardiomyocytes*, words whose tang I savored, not understanding. I liked to make up sentences anyway: The COX-1 cells upregulate the C tail of the heterodimer. The neonatal mouse pups are rinsed and pelleted. The PI is visualized at 25,000 rpm. None of these sentences make much sense, but Theresa and I both remember a time when I accidentally said something true.

For a long time, I did not think Theresa's kind of science had anything to do with this book. Theresa is a pharmacologist, not a molecular geneticist. She studies the proteins that genes encode. Her field is cell signaling; her specialty is G-protein mediated signal transduction, though in recent years she has begun to study heart cells too. All this translates, in my brain at least, to "the way cells talk to each other." I was more interested in chromosomes, in what they meant to people, in the metaphors I could make. But then, in August of 2006, I went to the triennial World Down Syndrome Conference, where I saw a neuroscientist named William Mobley talk about Down syndrome. His work raises the possibility—however distant—of a pharmacological approach to Down syndrome. Not a cure, or a wand, but a possible way to help the cells talk to each other, and perhaps to improve cognitive function overall.

If you had told me, when I first met Theresa, that I would be attending a conference on Down syndrome in British Columbia, while she took our kids off to the East Coast on vacation, so I could research a nonfiction book about our family—well, let's just say it would have seemed approximately as likely as having a career in systems engineering or international finance. But in 2006, the conference seemed worth the trouble. I packed my laptop, a file box of notes, and the few shirts and pants not torn or stained by cooking oil or solvents, then got in the ancient Subaru and headed up I-5 towards Vancouver.

In the plaza outside the convention center, parents stood around between sessions, name badges draped from their necks. Mine said GEORGE ESTREICH, USA. Some of the parents were accompanied by children with Down syndrome; some of the older children were presenters. We all milled around, mixing with the tourists who disembarked from the massive cruise ship docked alongside the Convention Center. It was like being in a country where Down syndrome was ordinary. There were the Down Syndrome Ambassadors, Canadians with Down syndrome who filed into the ballroom before each morning's plenary session; they wore matching, monogrammed Polarfleece vests. The peaceable kingdom of the chromosome, where the scientists and parents and children, the bisomic and the trisomic, sit down together.

I saw William Mobley's presentation in one of the morning plenary sessions. Mobley is a rangy, gray-haired neuroscientist, with the confident manner of people who are successful and tall. He works at Stanford University, and he is funded by the Down Syndrome Research and Treatment Foundation, a nonprofit that focuses basic research on cognitive problems. His model system is the mouse. It is one of the many surreal facts of our modern world that you can engineer mice to have Down syndrome. They have partial trisomies of chromosome 16—a mouse's sixteenth chromosome shares many genes with a human's twenty-first—and, as a result, they differ in predictable ways. They have smaller brains than regular mice, they exhibit many of the same anatomical features, and they take longer to do mazes. (Underwater mazes, as it turns out. My first thought: Mice can *swim?*)

To say that a mouse "has" Down syndrome is, in many ways, absurd. Mice may be able to swim, but they cannot, like Karen Gaffney, one of the speakers at the conference, swim around Alcatraz Island, then talk with confidence to a large crowd about what that felt like, then link the description of that experience to stories of growing up with Down syndrome, then conclude with a clear message of equality and inclusion. Neither do mice have friends, jobs, or Individual Education Plans. But they are mammals, with nervous systems much like ours. Therefore, it is possible to study cognition on two levels at once: in the maze, and under the microscope.

Mobley's research was focused on a normal phenomenon called NGF transport. NGF—short for neurotrophic growth factor—is one of the thousands of molecules that flash across the gap between neurons, but it is less messenger than gardener: its job is to keep the neurons healthy. If the neurons don't get enough NGF, they atrophy. So in animals—mice or human beings—where NGF transport is reduced, then the neurons wither too. Since the neurons of people with Down syndrome are already impaired in structure, their atrophy simply makes a bad situation worse.

Mobley was speaking the familiar-unknown language of Theresa's grants: *synapse, cholinergic receptors, upregulation.* It was an odd, stereoscopic feeling, hearing the words in the context of Down syndrome. But what brought me up short were the movies. Moving pictures of molecules, NGF or otherwise, are an extremely recent innovation, but Mobley was apparently well funded enough to have them. He showed, first of all, a movie of NGF transport in the regular mice: a cloud of molecules zipping healthily across the synapse, like the best night of the Pleiades, a clear dark sky and the shooting stars coming down, one after another. And then he showed the movie of NGF transport in the trisomic mice.

It was a different picture entirely. A few molecules, moving more slowly. They made their way across the screen like stars falling through maple syrup. Later that night, the podium would be moved away, the chairs would be cleared from the ballroom floor, and the Down Syndrome Ambassadors and their parents and friends and siblings would all be dancing. But for now, we were looking at NGF.

It was like watching the pace of thought itself. I knew this was false, one more metaphor misapplied, and yet I couldn't help it. I felt bad for them, the molecules, they almost seemed lonely. *Idiotos*, the root of *idiot*, means "lonely one" or "solitary one"—a connection Down himself remarked upon—and I thought suddenly of a loneliness that went right down to the dendrites. A molecular loneliness. Then, with a start, I felt awful. When I'd gotten impatient with Laura, or the few times I'd lost it and yelled, I had been getting mad over something that, at the profoundest level, could not be helped. Her molecules were moving slower. But then, those were the days when my molecules were moving slower too.

Mobley also reported on the startling success of one of his colleagues, who had administered a drug called PTZ to the trisomic mice. When he tested the mice, their cognition had improved. They negotiated their mazes faster; they remembered the solution longer. There was sudden whispering in the room. Mobley had to clarify: there is now no drug for Down syndrome. In human beings, the seizures induced by

PTZ would outweigh any cognitive benefit. Since the PTZ discovery, other candidate drugs have shown promise. But because of the differences between human beings and mice, and because of the necessarily slow pace of clinical trials, a pill is a long way off. For now, I'm placing my bets on a well-written IEP.

But there in the ballroom, absorbing Mobley's work, I felt a slow dawning, a synaptic shift of my own. All along I had been focused on the chromosome, but as Theresa told me early on, it's not just the genes, it's gene expression. It's the proteins, which the genes code for. For the first time that idea became real, and at the same time my idea of Down syndrome shifted. Whatever realizations I had come to and written, whatever progress I had made in understanding the chromosome as a script of inclusion, not separation, some trace of its monolithic nature had stayed with me. I think that, on some level, I will always see the chromosome as both imposing and microscopic. It is the doorway we all walked through, into another life.

But in the lens of Mobley's research, the chromosome seemed as ordinary as Laura. It was simply a collection of genes. Those genes coded for proteins. Some of the proteins mattered more than others. It was a matter of increments, not fates. It was a matter of molecules. If the promise of Mobley's research is fulfilled, then Down syndrome may become partially treatable, in the way that depression or ADHD is treatable: a pharmacological approach could become an adjunct to therapy. Not a wand, but a tool.

I looked around the ballroom. Seeing the faces around me, I saw the best reply to Down's mistake: the children looked like their parents. They looked like each other too, but it was clear that their true brothers and sisters were theirs by blood, not diagnosis. They were, to use Down's phrase, a part of the great human family. On my most hopeful days, on the days when my own molecules are up to speed, I think more people will come to share this perspective: that the diagnosis will be a footnote to individuality, and not the other way around;

that stories of ordinary lives will come to replace the tragedies and fables still accepted as truth; and that Laura will live in a world where she seems as ordinary to others as she does to us.

March 2007

We sit together at the low table in the children's room of the library, coloring the Xeroxed sheets set out for the children. Pumpkins at Halloween, turkeys at Thanksgiving, generic sleighs at Christmas, flowers in springtime, the round of the child's world, emblem by emblem, dark definite lines to color in. She's getting better at coloring. She used to grip the crayon in her fist, roughing in vast areas of color, and now she holds the crayon like a pencil. She stays inside the lines, for the most part. I write on the blank back of the sheets, scribbling new ideas and chapter outlines and notes on tone. Roman numerals, arrows, fragments. At home I type them out: *prenatal diagnosis, Earlswood, transhuman.* On the other side: *barnyard, teddy bear, beaver.*

We're in the fast-forward part of life. Theresa got tenure. Penny died, after thirteen years. For weeks afterwards I expected to see her when I walked in the door. We have a guinea pig now, which Ellie finally got after extensive negotiations. She named the pig "Poppy," after spending a long time considering "Daisy." Poppy has a custom cage, made of wire mesh and leftover trim from the old house. I slip cartoons about Poppy into Ellie's lunch box. He has a friend, Alien, a potato-shaped blob with two big eyes. Ellie's in fifth grade now, going into middle school next year; I'm glad she hasn't quite outgrown the cartoons.

Laura's near the end of her first year of kindergarten, and despite the predictable bumps at the beginning, things have gone well. She's in the regular full-day class; an aide divides her time between Laura and the two or three other kids on IEPs. Most of the time, Laura doesn't want the help. She wants to sit with the other kids; they have welcomed her, more than I ever thought possible, and since she feels like one of the class, she does her best to keep up. She can write the alphabet, count to ten, and write her name. She's not at grade level and will never be, but she's doing well.

She's beginning to read. I'd seen a presentation at WDSC 2006 by Patricia Oelwein, the Down syndrome reading specialist, who emphasized that people with Down syndrome tend to be visual learners, and that whole-word recognition should precede phonics. We got Oelwein's book. We began making flash cards: *dog, cat, vacuum, Laura, Mom, Dad, Ellie.* She's up to thirty-five words now. It's not hard to imagine her reading, one day, at the sixth-grade level most Americans read at. Maybe she'll read this book too. If she can, I will ask her what she thinks of it. If she can't, I'll tell her about it, in whatever way makes sense to her most. The explanation, if necessary, will be redundant. She will understand, better than I ever can, the way people with Down syndrome are seen.

Now and then, I am surprised to discover that I have a daughter with Down syndrome. I turn mental corners and there it is: Whoa! A mild surprise, a ghost of the original shock, though what once felt like lightning on a hilltop is now more like static in a dry season, little sparks from a doorknob or the touch of a child's hand.

I knew nothing about Down syndrome except that it was bad, and that it meant Laura was different from me. I no longer believe the first—Down syndrome is simply Laura's way of being human. As for the second: Laura *is* different, but the differences are superficial. This may seem an odd assertion, since the extra chromosome pervades her, and its effects texture our days. And yet these altered forms, eye and face and word, have come to contain and absorb what I know of love. Or love learned to alter itself, to accommodate the forms. She is no less my daughter, no less a person, for having an extra chromosome.

When she was in the ICU, choking on debris in her ventilator tube, and I stood in the hallway watching the child's palette of her crashing vitals—blue, lavender, green—I didn't feel much, not even fear, which is only to say that *feeling* is too small a word to describe the change that had already begun. I don't mean that I became, in any way, a different person. I am much the same. But I was beginning to understand the paradox of Down syndrome: that a child who embodied difference, eye and heart and cell, exposed the deep similarities implicit in raising any child. Our second daughter taught us the responsibilities we had accepted, when we chose to have our first. Laura's chromosome count taught me that every child is a genetic risk; her heart defect taught me that the risk is mortal; and years later, remembering an infant I did not know, I learn—again—that it is not only the chromosome, but our response to it, that shapes the contours of a life. Every tube, every wire, the violent nurture of surgery and the gentler nurture of feeding therapy, all working towards the clear pronunciation of a word: these hinged on the belief that her life was worth saving in the first place, then nurturing to its fullest potential. Everything we have done, teaching her to eat, to speak, every act of ambassadorship and interpretation, presumes the uncomplicated belief that her life is radically, democratically valuable. If we did not, on some level, believe that, we would not even have taken her home.

Tokyo, 1945

In the summer of 2006, I got a phone call from my mom. She had gotten a fund-raising letter from WNET, the PBS television station in New York, accompanied by a call for memories, and she wanted to write something and send it in.

The occasion was Ken Burns's new documentary *The War.* According to the letter, Burns "realized that every day—as more of our fathers and mothers, grandfathers and grandmothers succumb to the passage of time—<u>you and I are losing a connection to the *personal* memories and deeds of this generation</u>." Enclosed with the letter was a piece of lined paper, headlined "Share a memory from the World War II era"; it continued, "Please feel free to share any memory from roughly September 1939 to September 1945." There were bulleted thought questions on the back of the page:

- How did life change for you as a result of the war?
- What are the most vivid memories you have of the war years?
- What hardships did you face? Did you plant a Victory Garden?

The letter was encouraging ("<u>you</u> may be a goldmine of memories about World War II"), so my mom typed something up and sent it in. She sent me what she wrote, along with a copy of the fund-raising letter. Stuck on the document was a blue-gray Post-It: "Dear George, Here it is. Let me know what you think of it. Love, Mom."

I'd been asking about the war for years. If I'd known sending her a form letter would have worked better, I would've sent something on Channel Thirteen letterhead long ago.

In her essay, she describes the firebombing of Tokyo:

> In the evening of March 10th . . . hundreds of B-29s (333 planes according to the record) came over Tokyo and dropped countless incendiary bombs over the downtown area. I was in the shelter throughout the ordeal shivering from both cold and fear. When the raid was finally over, I climbed the ladder to the roof to look at the direction of the downtown . . . I would never forget what I saw there: black, purple, red smoke clouds were moving slowly in coils covering the horizon. That night more than a hundred thousand civilians were killed in the fire. My maternal grandmother was one of them.

The air raids continue, and on May twenty-fifth the bombs fall close to the house. Her mother gives her a scarf to cover her eyes and nose and mouth against the dust. In a beautiful passage that remembers the unimaginable, she describes what she sees the next morning:

> The following day, I went to see the expanse of the burned area. Stacks of tatami mats were still burning, and there was an overwhelming burning smell. With it of all things, was a sweet smell of perfume floating from the destroyed perfume factory on the other side of the railroad tracks. Some places which I had till then thought were in distance, like the train station, appeared right there in a short walking distance.

Soon afterwards, Japan surrendered. My mother was outside Shinjuku Station when the emperor's voice came on the radio. "[As] we listened to the speech standing in the hot sun among destruction, we all cried tears running down our cheeks. Yet we all felt relieved after that. We were now able to sleep without worrying about air-raid sirens, and my family and I waited for my brother to come home." She adds that the emperor's voice, which no one outside the palace had ever heard before, "was not very impressive."

Her family waits a long time for her brother to return, her beloved brother, ten years older than she. Even when I was young, I knew about her brother, that his loss had left her devastated and unconsoled. But I did not know anything more until I read what my mom wrote for Channel Thirteen:

At the beginning we heard from him by postcards. In one of them he wrote a haiku poem, but a couple of words were blotted out by black ink and we could not read them. Obviously they had been censored. My parents carefully wiped off the black ink till we could decipher the words, which were "one coconut." My father surmised that the censor did not want us, his family back home, to find out where he was. Coconut suggested south seas where palm trees grew and not north. "Silly," my father muttered, "We all knew which direction he was going."

As time went on there was no more news from him and we suspected the worst. Then one day a man who'd been with my brother visited us. I wasn't home and so I did not meet him. What he said was that he'd been with my brother in a place called Manokwari in New Guinea until a day before the place was attacked. So he was able to come back, but my brother who had remained there another day to take care of some business was killed. It was June 1944. When I heard about it, I became more angry than sad. I went into my room and shut the door. Just one day! If he had evacuated one day earlier, he would have been home!

My younger brother then came to my room bringing me a cup of warm sugar water from Mother. Because of the acute food shortage, everything was on ration. We had not seen meat or fish for sometime and rice we received on ration was in a very small amount. So to increase the volume, my mother added a lot of water when she cooked rice into gruel.

We used to eat sweet potatoes for snacks, but now potato was part of our main meal, and for snacks if we did have snacks, we were given sugar water. That is if there were any sugar in the house. And now, my younger brother was bringing me precious sugar water to comfort me. I took the cup from him but could not bring myself to drink it. How could I drink sugar water when I now knew for sure my brother had died! With all the force I threw the cup against the wall.

PBS loved it, and two passages were selected for a documentary called *New York War Stories*. When my mom visited in the fall, she brought the DVD with her. We all sat in the family room and watched the documentary. Laura cuddled with Theresa, and drifted off to sleep. Ellie watched with us. When my mom's part came on, we heard an actor speaking. My mom shrugged. "I guess they didn't like my voice," she said.

It was a good visit. My mom's writing was out in the world. Ellie was beginning to grasp what her grandmother had been through. I could *see* it sinking in, the way I have watched her, over the years, come to understand more and more of Laura's strange but real place in the world. Ellie is joined by chance and chromosome to these unimaginable lives, but she is somehow able to imagine them. Once, as I tried in my fumbling too-detailed way to explain what my book was about, she said, "It's like once you decide someone's different, then all you notice is differences."

We have had to imagine Laura; Ellie has had to imagine the world. Ellie began with what seemed a pure shrug of acceptance, and has gradually come to understand what she accepted; and we, her parents, have learned the meaning of the acceptance we talked about. In the middle is Laura, who could care less. She likes playing with my mom, whom she calls "Ba." In Laura, *Ba*—derived from *Obachama*, which means grandmother in Japanese—means Grandma. Since *Ba* is easy to say, she uses the word for Theresa's mom too.

Not long ago, we visited my mom in New Jersey. When we had settled in and been overfed to my mother's satisfaction, she got out the colored blocks I used to play with, and set them up for Laura. Each has a letter on it, from the hiragana alphabet; she had gotten them, I think, hoping they would help me and my sisters learn Japanese. She set them in towers for Laura, as she used to for Ellie, and many years before, for me. Like Ellie, like me, Laura gleefully smacked the towers down, saying *zoom!* I got out the album for Ellie, and showed her the photo, held in place by crisp black triangles: George in a New York apartment, swiping at the piled blocks, laughing when they fall down. I'm a year old in the picture. My hair is wispy; my features, more recognizably Japanese.

"Awww," said Ellie.

In the beginning, after Laura's diagnosis, it was easy to think that my mom was in denial and I was facing facts. It's probably more accurate to say that we were going through a similar process, but that I was more fluent at disguising it. We were talking about Laura, Down syndrome, chromosomes, and Mongols, but that language expressed older, more ordinary things: family history, the old battles between a mother and son too much alike, the aftermath of my father's death, the trauma of a war at once distant and immediate. Things that could not be helped.

Reading my mother's stories about the war did not undo the difficulties and the years between us. But to glimpse, for the first time, what she had gone through was the beginning of understanding. I write this out of love, and out of an understanding that at a certain point one simply moves on. We do not have a choice about what was said, but we have a choice about what to say next. The argument between us, the haze of resentment, blame, shock, and anger, seems distant now. It was never worth winning anyway. We have moved from truce to truce; I write this in hopes of peace.

Once, in first grade, Laura brought home a pink paper bowl; the rim of the bowl was hole-punched all the way around, and blue strings were tied to the holes, so they dangled. It was meant to look like a Portuguese man-of-war. Laura held it overhead, shook the strings, and said, "Thow."

Thow. We don't always get what Laura means, but this time I knew: she meant *shower*. The bowl was the showerhead, and the blue strings were water. This is something to make a poet's heart proud: a lightning, performative little haiku, a metaphor, a rewriting of the object with imagination.

We live from haiku to haiku, mostly verbless. We communicate in telegrams. We speak Laura, and we adjust without really thinking about it. In the grocery store, if I say, "Laura, can you get me five limes," she takes the plastic bag, reaches up towards the limes, counts five ("wan, two, thee, f'no, vaff"). If she were to say, "Hey Dad, here are the five limes you asked for," I'd be speechless. Though she understands me, her speech lags behind her comprehension.

It's not all haiku and limes. Laura can be a royal pain, and on my bad days she and I often set up the sort of feedback loop parents hate but fall into anyway: I get impatient, I yell, she yells back. She loves Ellie and worships Ellie, and Ellie loves her, but they also bicker, and she pesters Ellie, for no good reason, as little sisters do. But this is life. This is, in every sense, normal.

She's been reading for some time, though by most standards she's probably more of a prereader than anything. Like many children with Down syndrome, she does best with sight words, not phonics: she recognizes the shapes, but as of this writing (at the age of eight) she is not quite ready to sound out words by reading the letters. But she can probably read around a hundred words. When I began, I was inordinately proud of the number of words, and immediately set to teaching her a vocabulary as impractical as her original vocabulary in Sign: zoo animals, colors, and so on. At a certain point I realized she was living in a world of nouns. I was helped to this realization by her Life Skills teacher, Mo Ruzek, who gently emphasized the importance of the forgotten words, the little ones, *the*, *said*, *it*, *is*, *with*, without which we live in a telegram world. We shifted away from piling up the gold coins of vocabulary. We began to work on reading sentences, something we will be doing for quite a while. Laura likes using the laptop, probably because it stops me from writing. I close the latest draft, open DOCUMENT 1, and type, in 48 point Times, sentences like this:

Laura is a girl

I like to swim

Mom is at work

I like to play with Ellie

Dad is a dinosaur

I can eat a house

She giggles, she gets the joke. I get a lot of mileage out of saying the wrong thing, *Laura can eat a car*, just the way I did with Ellie.

When Ellie was learning to write, she used to capitalize *I* whenever it occurred. She assumed, since it was capitalized by itself, that it should be capitalized elsewhere too. It is the kind of error that reveals intelligence, a mind solving a problem, and I see it now when Laura reads. She gets a lot of things right, but her mistakes are as meaningful as her successes. For *green* she says *yellow*; for *hat* she says *bat*; for *book*, *door*; for *door*, *chair*; for *Laura*, *I*. She is moving beyond the sight-word. She is recognizing word-shapes, treating each word as a *kanji*, a single character, a pictogram: but even so she is already beginning to break down the brushstrokes, to see patterns. She is processing, analyzing, *thinking*.

To see Laura reading—to see her press a finger to the word *swim* and say "dtim," or *Dad* and say "Dat," to *dog* and say "daw"—is a complex experience. I am proud of her, of course, in precisely the same way I am proud of Ellie, whenever Ellie achieves something new. The old question *what can you expect from a child with Down syndrome* now seems roughly as silly as the question *what can you expect from a child*: you have to know which child you're talking about. If you have two kids—a mathlete and a jock, say—you don't hold one child to the other's standards. The presence of Down syndrome sharpens this point, but the principle is the same: we're happy when Laura reads *swim*, and we're happy when Ellie solves the hardest quadratic equation on that day's homework, but the expectations, like the children, are not interchangeable.

What will become of them? What will happen, as Ellie becomes a teenager, then an adult? Will Laura follow her to college? Will she live with us? Will Ellie live close by, or far away? What will happen, after we are gone? We don't know. We save, prepare, forge the links we need to forge, keep our expectations high. Beyond that, we cannot say, but then, we cannot say with any child. Anything can happen. We do what we would do if they had the same number of chromosomes: we try to prepare them for the future we do not know.

When we walked into an exam room, eight years ago, we learned that Laura had Down syndrome. For a long time, I thought we had learned a difficult fact. But we were really at the beginning of a conversation.

Dr. E.—Kevin—told us, in a sentence that embodied friendship and consolation and hope, that "these children come to the families most able to take care of them." What have we done but to make that sentence ours? We needed to parse it, word by word: we needed to learn again what *children* meant, to see how this child differed from *these children*, to see that *these children* were not so different from others. We needed to learn what *family* meant, and *able*, we had to open *able* and *ability* wide enough to admit both of our daughters, both able, both loved. And although the fact we were there to learn—*Laura does have Down syndrome*—felt like a fate, a sentence whose term was fixed, we have come to understand it as a simple declaration, an utterance whose meaning was open. It was up to us.

As we discovered this, we became the people our doctor described. Though we were haunted by an old story, we knew enough to begin a new one; and though his words were not the ones we would have chosen, we have learned how to make them true.

November 2009

It's Monday, and Laura doesn't want to go to school. It's 7:55 A.M., and we have to be out the door in five minutes. She's a little bit sniffly, but it's intermittent/clear, and she slept well. No fever, plenty of energy.

"Laura," I say. "Time for school. Get your shoes on."

"No," she says. "Sick."

"You're not sick," I say. "You're fine. Let's go."

"*Sick*," she says. Then: "Car."

"That's right," I tell her. "We have to go to the car. Now. So let's get your shoes on."

"No," she says. "*Car*." She pulls up her shirt, and I start to tell her to pull her shirt down, and then I see her pointing to the scar from her heart surgery.

"*Car*," she says, emphatically. "Sick." She thumps her chest.

"Laura," I say, trying not to laugh. "That's from long ago, when you were a little baby. That's all better now."

"Oh," she says.

"Shoes on," I say.

She grumbles but consents. Theresa and I take Laura to the car. Just before we pull into the drop-off zone for Jefferson School, I look back and see that Laura's clear, intermittent sniffle has gone nuclear and green.

"Maybe she should stay home," I say. "With the flu thing, she'll probably get sent home anyhow."

"It's not the flu," says Theresa. "But you're probably right."

We drop Theresa off at work ("Bye, Mum," says Laura, chipper as ever) and head back home to take Ellie to middle school. Ellie looks at Laura. The sniffle is gone. Laura has a smile as big as Iowa.

"*Someone* seems sprightly today," Ellie says.

"Yeah," I say. "But I figured I'd keep her home, just to be on the safe side."

Laura has a plan. "*Star Wars?*" she says. "Pod race?" *The Phantom Menace* is her current favorite; given a choice, she'd rerun the Tatooine pod race all morning.

"No TV," I tell her. "Homework first. We have to do your reading, and you have to practice your spelling words." For actual sick, with flu, fever, and the works, I'd set up the *Star Wars*/Wiggles marathon. For sort-of-sniffly sick, though, it's homework and errands with Dad.

Laura looks disappointed.

"Feel better," she says.

Afterword
Marcia Day Childress

On soft, humid summer evenings, the pedestrian mall in Charlottesville, Virginia, comes alive. Brick-paved and lined with willow oaks whose dense canopy glows after dark with tiny white lights, the six-block mall is home to outdoor cafés, crafts vendors, live music, and a parade of people—young families, runners, gaggles of teens, pairs of elders, purposeful dog-walkers, strolling lovers. It's in this setting that I've seen, twice now, walking hand in hand and with eyes only for each other, a young man and young woman, both with Down syndrome.

I know nothing more than this about the couple's situation. But they—as individual members of our community and as partners—represent to me a new perspective on the genetic condition identified in the nineteenth century by John Langdon Down and eponymously named. Until recent decades, *mongoloid* was a descriptor given persons with Down syndrome, institutionalization or domestic sequestration was the preferred way of handling them, and shame and pity were emotions their presence aroused in families and bystanders. This couple—their apparent independence as well as their togetherness—signals a momentous shift.

So too does *The Shape of the Eye*, George Estreich's memoir about raising his second daughter, Laura, who has Down syndrome. Estreich details a very different story of Down syndrome from the traditional textbook tale of etiology, pathophysiology, signs and symptoms, diagnosis, clinical course and complications, and prognosis. While embedding within his story the sobering medical, historical, and social narratives of this genetic condition, replete with connections to the eugenics movement and to ideas about western biomedicine's progress toward human perfection (or, at least, toward the elimination of significant abnormality), Estreich's memoir embraces all aspects of the lived experience of rearing a child with this particular genetic makeup. His story of Down syndrome both greatly expands upon and effectively counterbalances the clinical tale.

And updates it. Page by page, *The Shape of the Eye* demonstrates very real possibilities for significant quality of life now for persons who have Down syndrome, and so departs markedly from past biomedical appraisals and social stigmatization. Laura has already attained physical and cognitive developmental milestones well beyond the dim prospects catalogued in twentieth-century medical texts for children with this genetic profile. Since a biomedical perspective may chiefly problematize a condition, parsing the ways in which affliction signals defect, damage, loss, and "less than," medicalized responses to Down syndrome, including the institutionalization and social marginalization of affected children and the abortion of fetuses with trisomy 21 following prenatal genetic screening, have long limited our ability to understand how such persons might live, learn, and socialize. If we now know more about the capabilities of persons with Down syndrome, we must also thank medicine and its practitioners for devising ways to treat the condition's physical complications, including serious heart problems, and thus for helping to extend average life expectancy well beyond the twenty-five years estimated in 1980. Similarly, we owe debts to other health care and educational specialists—from occupational and speech therapists to experts in nutrition, schooling, life-skills instruction, and job training—for developing interventions that better enable persons with Down syndrome to lead bountiful lives and participate meaningfully in our communities.

If disability is a lens through which society sees persons with Down syndrome, changing norms, laws, and practices around disability now ask us to acknowledge *difference*, not *defect*, in these individuals. The thrust of disability advocacy today is to include persons like Laura to every extent possible in the mainstream of our common life. While some in our society may yet stigmatize and harbor moral judgments about persons with Down syndrome, their numbers are dwindling. Collective attitudes and practices are shifting toward accommodation and appreciation both of these individuals' innate and tutored capabilities and, indeed, their gifts for affection, loyalty, industry, and friendship. *The Shape of the Eye* invites us to see the manifold ways in which Laura—and her family—can flourish in our midst. The story of Laura's upbringing also shows how health care, social service, and educational resources help to make her flourishing possible—and with this book her father pleads an eloquent, if implicit, case for sustained support of such resources, public and private.

Above all, *The Shape of the Eye* personalizes Down syndrome, bringing a condition abstracted in the medical literature into the full dimensionality of one family's life. It's brave of George Estreich to make what has befallen his family so public, trusting of him to let an unknown audience second-guess the family's choices. Because he's opened his home and heart in this memoir, we are privileged to witness in chaotic, heart-wrenching, joyous detail what it means to have and to love a child with Down syndrome. Writing *The Shape of the Eye* afforded Estreich the chance to take the measure of this unexpected turn and the impact it has had on him and Theresa, on their marriage, on their older daughter Ellie, and the life they've made in the years since Laura was born.

Estreich's memoir joins a growing library of contemporary caregiver narratives that chronicle serious illnesses or conditions not simply as personal challenges or medical (mis)adventures for the afflicted individuals but also as emotionally complicated, socioeconomically daunting occasions of being-in-the-world that fundamentally reorder family life, reconfigure relationships, rewrite family history. Such narratives abound—among the better known published memoirs of caregiving are Robert and Peggy Stinson's *The Long Dying of Baby Andrew* (Little Brown,1983), Alan Shapiro's brotherly remembrance *Vigil* (Chicago, 1997), Donald Hall's grieving poems in *Without* (Houghton Mifflin, 1998), John Bayley's *Elegy for Iris* (St. Martin's, 1999), Elizabeth Hall Hutner's sonnets in *Life with Sam* (Cavankerry, 2002), Rebecca Brown's alphabetical vignettes in *Excerpts from a Family Medical Dictionary* (Wisconsin, 2003), Brian Fies's graphic memoir *Mom's Cancer* (Abrams Image, 2006), Madge McKeithen's evocative essays in *Blue Peninsula* (Farrar, Straus & Giroux, 2006), Aaron Alterra's poignant *The Caregiver: A Life with Alzheimer's* (Cornell, 2008), and Michael Greenberg's impassioned *Hurry Down Sunshine* (Vintage, 2009). There is also Carol Levine's *Always on Call* (Vanderbilt, 2004), a superb collection that includes first-person essays by a variety of caregivers, Levine included ("The Loneliness of the Long-Term Caregiver").

In each caregiver's account, as in Estreich's, illness and caregiving inform and inflect everything inside the family circle, including whatever might constitute happiness and healing. Each narrative demonstrates that illness and caregiving are deeply intertwined in their expression, effects, and interpretation. If caregiver narratives model for us both how to give care and how to survive the burdens and losses of caregiving, many such stories also blaze the way toward living meaningfully with chronic vulnerability, challenge, or disability. In a society where biomedicine's successes account for a burgeoning population of persons whose chronic conditions and functional impairments require considerable caregiving by family and others, the caregiver's story is one to which we should all attend. Such a tale may one day become ours to tell.

Caregiver narratives about specific conditions—from prematurity to Alzheimer's dementia, from cancer to quadriplegia—are frequently read by persons for whom a family member's diagnosis has turned the world upside down and made caregiving their new way of life. Fellow travelers' stories can be touchstones in the caregiver's often-lonely journey. They may offer sage advice, model or caution against certain approaches to care, provide encouragement, instill hope. Almost always, they attest to the profound intersubjectivity and interdependency of those who give and receive care. Caregiver narratives also bring bioethics home, as it were, grounding ethical questions and decisions in the particularities and practicalities of the everyday, one person's illness or one domestic caregiving situation at a time.

Increasingly, caregiver stories are included in medical humanities or narrative medicine courses for physicians- and nurses-in-training, in hopes these accounts may acquaint young clinicians more thoroughly with their future patients' worlds and with the often-messy lives of families who will seek their services. Indeed, I see a place for *The Shape of the Eye* in my classrooms at the University of Virginia, in both the medical school, where I offer a literature and medicine elective for fourth-year medical students and in the English department, where undergraduates planning to enter the health professions take my course, *Narratives of Illness and Doctoring.*

As a caregiver memoir, *The Shape of the Eye* is radiant with human complexity and possibility. In her family, Laura is exceptional, to be sure, and her care and nurturing present obstacles George and Theresa never faced with Ellie. For Laura and her family, even supposedly straightforward developmental steps—wanting and learning to take food by mouth, for instance—are fraught with difficulty and require professional help. Family outings, marital tensions, and sibling relationships are all complicated by Laura's condition and needs. And accepting and loving Laura are made more difficult for her Japanese grandmother—George's mother—not only by the medicalizing of Laura's identity in infancy but also by her facial appearance (at once characteristic of Down syndrome and her Japanese heritage) and the racially derogatory *mongoloid* label.

As readers, we readily grasp that Laura's genetic makeup requires her family's attention, effort, and expense. We may marvel at their stamina and steadfastness in the face of a lifetime's challenges—medical, social, and economic. But, importantly, *The Shape of the Eye* reveals much of the family's life to be reassuringly ordinary—Ellie's and Laura's schooling, Theresa's academic career, George's writing and homefront responsibilities. Their story is so much more than an "illness narrative" (the book is remarkable too for being the story of a stay-at-home dad and, as such, another kind of social-modeling narrative for our time). But what may be most compelling about *The Shape of the Eye* is the way it both mainstreams and transcends Down syndrome, revealing in heartfelt detail how Laura's parents have come to know and love her, how they advocate for and work with her, how their daughter with this particular genetic makeup is every bit as human, quirky, and full of her own potential as her older sister Ellie.

Summer having given way to autumn, the crowd on our downtown mall at twilight is smaller now, café business sparser, pedestrians' paces brisker. I've not seen again that young couple, both with Down syndrome, walking hand in hand along the leaf-strewn bricks of the promenade. But I wonder whether Laura Estreich might one day stroll this space, and in whose company she'll walk, a visitor to the Charlottesville her parents knew a generation ago as University of Virginia students. I trust she'd feel safe and welcomed.

One night this October, watching HBO television, I happened upon the documentary film "Monica and David" about love that blossomed between two young adults with Down syndrome, their wedding, and the fragile balance of independence and support to be maintained as they embark on married life. Ali Codina's intimate and moving film about her cousin Monica's new life won Best Documentary Feature at the 2010 Tribeca Film Festival. Like *The Shape of the Eye*, "Monica and David" powerfully signals our society's new perspectives on Down syndrome. Both the book and the film will change minds, and hearts, about Down syndrome and the persons among us who happen to have it. Serendipity—the film is coming to Charlottesville this November, to a theater on the downtown mall, as part of the annual Virginia Film Festival. I wonder who I'll see there.

Marcia Day Childress is an associate professor of medical education and directs programs in humanities within the Center for Biomedical Ethics and Humanities at the University of Virginia's School of Medicine.

Acknowledgments

Thanks to the many who have read this book in manuscript, and whose friendship, suggestions, and encouragement have helped me along the way. Particular thanks must go to Edward Hardy, who encouraged me from the beginning of this project and read many, many words that never saw the light of day; to Michael McFee, for sustained encouragement, and for a detailed and insightful reading of a late draft; to Matt Yurdana, fellow poet, who cheered on the best parts of the book, while gently suggesting I might cut "maybe fifty pages" of duller bits; and to Tracy Daugherty, who supported the manuscript when its fortunes were dim, who urged me to persevere through one more draft, and whose insights on narrative helped me find a way through. Thanks also to Sara Gelser, Charles Goodrich, Anjali Jain, Jon Lewis, Lori Patel, Betsy Pohlman, and Marjorie Sandor, all of whom read early drafts or chapters and offered both perceptive commentary and support. Thanks, also, to the experts who took the time to answer my questions: Karina Aiberti, Christine Jepsen, Tom Markello, Marcia Van Riper, and Jennifer Wishart. A special thanks to SMU Press's outside readers, Lee Martin and Marcia Childress, and to Marcia especially for her thoughtful afterword.

I count myself lucky that my manuscript landed at SMU Press, and the main reason is my editor, Kathryn Lang. Kathryn is sharp-eyed for detail and structure, uncompromising about quality yet flexible about approach, and absolutely dedicated to her authors. Without her efforts, this book would still be a manuscript in a drawer, and for this I will be forever grateful. I also want to thank everyone at SMU Press:

George Ann Ratchford, for her work on marketing and design; Keith Gregory, the director of SMU Press; and everyone on SMU's Editorial Board for their support. Thanks also to Kellye Sanford for a beautiful cover design, and to Bob Fullilove for his thorough and thoughtful copyediting. (Any errors that remain are mine alone.)

Thanks also to the Oregon Literary Foundation, whose grant helped support the writing of this work, and to Caldera, which provided me with a quiet place to write—as did Tod Woodford, whose cabin was a welcome refuge in which to revise. Thanks to the editors of *Ambulatory Pediatrics*, who published brief excerpts from this book (in Vol. 8, No. 6). I presented other excerpts, in very different form, to a meeting of the Willamette Valley Down Syndrome Association (2003); at the World Down Syndrome Conference in Vancouver (2006); and at *Catching Fire*, a conference sponsored by the Spring Creek Project on Nature and the Sacred (2004).

Thanks to everyone who has helped Laura heal, grow, and learn over the years: our many friends, and Laura's, in Corvallis, Portland, and beyond; the doctors, nurses, and staff at Samaritan Family Medicine, Mid-Valley Children's Clinic, Good Samaritan Hospital, Doernbecher Children's Hospital, and Oregon Health Sciences University; the staff of the feeding clinic at the Children's Development and Rehabilitation Center; the therapists, staff, and coordinators from Benton County Early Intervention and Early Childhood Special Education; the teachers, administrators, and staff at Kindercare, Bates Hall, Dixie Developmental Preschool, Port Phillip Specialist School, and Jefferson Elementary School; the Willamette Valley Down Syndrome Association; and the staff, coordinators, and volunteers at Oregon State's IMPACT program. Some are named in the narrative, but all have our gratitude. (A few have preferred to remain anonymous. For that reason, I have changed some names and identifying details in the text.)

This is a book about family, and it could not have been written without the support of family, in every sense. Thanks to my sisters, Lisa

Estreich and Nina Estreich. Thanks to my wife's sisters, her brother, and their families—Bonnie and Pete Motel, Susan and Neil Margolis, Karen and Craig Peterson, and Mike and Mallika Filtz—and a special thanks to all of Laura's cousins, the "wolf pack" mentioned in the eleventh chapter: Amanda, Emma, Nathan, Randy, Mia, Owen, Katie, Ryan, and Eric. Thanks to Carole Filtz, my mother-in-law, for her love and support over the years, for being a terrific Grandma, and for taking care of Ellie and Laura on several occasions over the years, so that I could go off and write. And thanks to my mother, Ranko Estreich, for being a great Obachama, for sharing her stories in person and in her unpublished manuscripts, for the grace with which she has permitted me to write about her, and for teaching me, among many other things, the persistence required to finish a book.

Since this book already suggests what my wife and daughters mean to me, I'll spare everyone further embarrassment and focus on the book. My wife, Theresa Filtz, read countless drafts, made time for me to write, and allowed me to write about our life as a family. Laura didn't know I was writing about her at first, but knows there's a book about her now. I hope she'll read it one day.

A special thanks has to go to Laura's big sister, Ellie, who was entering kindergarten as I began this book and will have her learner's permit by the time it appears. She's been a patient child during the many hours when I was absorbed in this book, she read an early draft and gave me vital encouragement, and she's allowed me to write about her. But more than that, her initial reaction to Laura's diagnosis gives me hope: perhaps more people, like Ellie, will come to shrug at the diagnosis, and assume the fact of dignity, rather than the other way around. For all these reasons—but most of all, because Ellie is Ellie—this book is dedicated to her.

Notes

INTRODUCTION

p. xi   *"Laura does have Down syndrome"*: In the delivery of Laura's diagnosis, we were fortunate; but our experience is not necessarily typical. In 2005 Brian Skotko, then a medical student at Harvard University, published a study in *Pediatrics*. In it, he reports the results of a survey of over nine hundred American mothers on their experience of postnatal diagnosis. For all, finding out that a child had Down syndrome was anxiety-producing, as one would expect. But anxiety correlated strongly with the way the news was conveyed. If Down syndrome was described in negative ways, the mother's anxiety level rose; if positive aspects were illuminated, mothers were reassured. None of this is surprising. But Skotko also found that negative and outdated portrayals still abounded. Under the aegis of medical fact, some parents were told an old story of incapability, of children who could not "make change for the bus" (75), or who would always be a burden. Skotko concludes by recommending, among other things, that doctors try to convey a balanced portrait of the condition, not glossing over the possible problems, but also emphasizing the child first (74–76). Descriptions like this exist—and as Skotko found, doctors and nurses were more than glad to have them. But they are not yet the norm.

ARRIVAL

p. 7   *some people with Down syndrome do attend college:* See, for example, the profile of Katie Apostolides in the *New York Times* article "'Just a Normal Girl,'" by Leslie Kaufman, November 5, 2006. Accessed at http://www.nytimes.com/2006/11/05/education/edlife/downs.html.

A CHILD FIRST

p. 17   *In a parable of acceptance:* Kingsley, "Welcome to Holland."

p. 18   *the roses, the angels . . . the rhetoric of Holland:* Given the association of Holland and tulips, one would expect tulips. But roses, in my experience at least, are more common.

p. 18   *"I wanted people to say congratulations":* in Stray-Gundersen, *Babies with Down Syndrome,* 56.

p. 18   *"When the doctors told us":* in Stray-Gundersen, *Babies with Down Syndrome,* 55.

p. 18   *"My daughter is going on two":* in Stray-Gundersen, *Babies with Down Syndrome,* 60.

p. 19   *no Internet, nothing:* As a Web history of disability reports, "In both New York and New Jersey, parents looked for support by placing advertisements in the local newspaper: 'Are there any other parents out there who have a retarded child? Would you be interested in meeting and talking about this with another parent?'" Accessed at http://www.mncdd.org/parallels/five/5a/2.html.

p. 20   *and then we would mourn her:* In 2001 the life expectancy was about fifty-five. It was a long time before I thought to look at the publication date on the book, which was 1985. But in those days, it was easy to believe the worst.

BORDER

p. 45   *For this reason, clinicians depend on the NG tube:* Christine Jepsen, interview by author, Eugene, OR, December 13, 2001.

p. 47   *a New York Times article:* Ellen Barry, "A Place to Go When a Child Really Refuses Food," August 23, 2007. Accessed at http://www.nytimes.com/2007/08/23/nyregion/23eating.html.

THIS IS EATING

p. 59   *in the United States, it is Down syndrome, not Down's syndrome:* In the UK, the apostrophe is customary.

ECHO

p. 67   *a twenty-nine page booklet:* Sloan, *To Mend a Broken Heart.*

A COMPLEX SWEETNESS

p. 133   *"sweet":* This belief is ubiquitous: I found it in family medical guides, books about the Human Genome Project, and yellowing monographs retrieved from library storage. In a 1928 book entitled *Mongolism*, Kate Brousseau, an American asylum superintendent, writes: "Unlike infants of other types, Mongols are not given to fits of rage, are not ill-tempered, and are rarely destructive. They are usually good-natured, cheerful, affectionate, easily amused and frequently very shy in the presence of strangers. . . . Good humor and affectionate disposition appear to be characteristic of Mongolism" (122–23). Clemens Benda's 1943 monograph, *Mongolism and Cretinism*, holds that

"Mongoloid children, if treated well, are lovable little creatures full of affection and tenderness" (61). More recently, in the popular parenting guide *What to Expect the First Year*, we are told, after a long list of defects, that children with Down syndrome "are usually . . . very sweet and lovable" (644). And *Caring for Your Baby and Young Child: Birth to Age 5* by the American Academy of Pediatrics, after asserting that "most eventually are able to feed and dress themselves and to be toilet-trained," offers the consolation that "for all its difficulties, raising a child with Down syndrome can be deeply rewarding. Children with this condition are usually loving and openly affectionate, and will thrive if nurtured and loved in return" (634).

The "happy" stereotype comes from parents too. Notably, Dr. William Sears, parent of a son with Down syndrome and author: "What they may lack academically, these babies make up socially. Like all children, Down Syndrome babies have good and bad days. But, in general, these babies are affectionate and just plain happy. Many share constant hugs and kisses and radiate a generally carefree attitude. Their giving and caring attitudes are so contagious that those around these babies wonder who is really normal. There is indeed an up side to Down babies." Accessed at http://www.askdrsears.com/html/10/T107400.asp.

WRITERS AND FAMILIES

p. 148   *"JJMCP, JJMCP":* For the record, my mother denies having said this.

p. 149   ***"The multiple phenotypes that make up Down syndrome":*** Griffiths et al., *Introduction to Genetic Analysis*, 261–62.

p. 150   *in the mild to moderate range:* See, for example, the "Down Syndrome Fact Sheet" at http://www.ndss.org. See also Chahira Kozma, MD, "What Is Down Syndrome?" in Stray-Gundersen, *Babies with Down Syndrome,* 23.

p. 150   *rapidly approaching fifty:* "Of 17,897 people reported to have Down's syndrome, median age at death increased from 25 years in 1983 to 49 years in 1997, an average increase of 1.7 years per year studied." Quanhe Yang, Sonja A. Rasmussen, and J. M. Friedman, "Mortality Associated with Down's syndrome in the USA from 1983 to 1997: A Population-Based Study," *Lancet* 359, no. 9311 (2002): 1019.

THE LABYRINTH OF NORMAL

p. 157   *the labyrinth of Normal:* This is my take on a paradox noted by Michael Bérubé, in *Life as We Know It*: "On the one hand, we didn't want to measure Jamie [Bérubé's son] against normal children . . . on the other hand, we had no other scale to go by than that of 'normal' children. . . . It wasn't long before we realized that this paradox would be with us for the rest of our lives" (116).

For a discussion of the contradictory uses of the word "normal" in medical contexts, see Phillip V. Davis and John G. Bradley, "The Meaning of Normal," *Perspectives in Biology and Medicine* 40, no 1 (1996): 68–77.

p. 161   *"not black," "obliquely placed," "a slight dirty-yellowish tinge":* Down, "Observations on an Ethnic Classification of Idiots," in *Mental Affections,* 214.

p. 161   *Slanted language pervades:* In *Cracking the Genome: Inside the Race to Unlock Human DNA,* for example, we learn that "in addition to mental retardation, Down syndrome children suffer congenital heart disease, increased risk of leukemia, early-onset Alzheimer's disease, and scores of other developmental problems" (214). The author, Kevin Davies, is a founding editor of *Nature Genetics*. In a college-level text entitled *Bioethics and the New Embryology: Springboards for Debate*, the syndrome is described as "a malformation . . . caused by an extra copy of chromosome 21 in each cell. People with an extra copy of this very small chromosome suffer from mental retardation, the absence of a nasal bone, heart defects, a characteristic slanting of the eyes, and often the closure of the intestine" (23). The description is on a blue-shaded page entitled "Birth Defects." How "a characteristic slanting of the eyes" produces suffering is not explained.

p. 161   ***Life expectancy is underestimated:*** On life expectancy, see Ridley, *Genome*, quoted below; see also Anthony Griffiths et al., *Introduction to Genetic Analysis*, discussed in the previous chapter.

p. 161   ***Medical problems are exaggerated in severity and frequency:*** Many of the features of Down syndrome occur only rarely; most can be treated. In *Bioethics and the New Embryology*, cited above, "the closure of the intestine" is described as occurring "often" (23); according to Mark Selikowitz (in *Down Syndrome: The Facts*), duodenal atresias occur "in about 10 to 15 percent of infants with Down syndrome" (80). The condition is operable. By the terms of the description in *Bioethics*, every child born with Down syndrome has a heart defect; the actual occurrence is "about 40 to 45 percent," and these defects range greatly in severity (Chahira Kozma, MD, "Medical

Concerns and Treatments," in Stray-Gundersen, *Babies with Down Syndrome*, 65).

p. 161   ***The idea of tragedy, whether through financial ruin or the misery of siblings, is common:*** See *Your Genetic Destiny: Know Your Genes, Secure Your Health, Save Your Life* (2001), by the medical geneticist Aubrey Milunsky:

> Trisomy 21 or Down syndrome is evidenced by mental retardation and typical facial and other features (see Table 3.1). More than 85 percent of children born with this syndrome survive at least one year, and more than 50 percent live more than fifty years. Premature aging, with an increased frequency of early Alzheimer's disease, is common. Nevertheless, the average life expectancy of a person affected with Down syndrome now exceeds 60 years, given advances in the surgical correction of heart defects and in the treatment of common infections. The relatively long life expectancy has meant that brothers and sisters are almost invariably left with the burden of caring for those with Down syndrome. If there are no siblings, or none willing to take on their care, the State almost always ends up with this responsibility. (33)

For an earlier example, see *Human Genetics: A Modern Synthesis* (Boston: Jones and Bartlett, 1990), where the description of Down syndrome (in the chapter "Chromosomes: Normal and Abnormal") is a curious paradox: it does not describe Down syndrome. The author, Gordon Edlin, writes: "The risk that a woman will bear a Down child increases markedly past age thirty-five. . . . For that reason, all physicians (because of possible legal action) now recommend amniocentesis for all pregnant women of age thirty-five or older" (42).

As in Milunsky's account, longer life is the *source* of tragedy:

> With modern medical care, the life expectancy of a person having Down syndrom [*sic*] is now forty years or more. Because Down children ultimately exhaust both the financial and the emotional resources of their families, most of them are eventually placed in public institutions that are often crowded, understaffed, and underfunded. The plight of Down syndrome adults and other mentally deficient persons who have been committed to institutions is particularly tragic. However, with early physical therapy and continued encouragement by family and therapists, some of those having Down syndrome can achieve a measure of independence in living. Still, most couples who learn that the pregnant mother will bear a Down or other severely handicapped child elect to abort the pregnancy. (42–43)

By 1990 deinstitutionalization was well under way, parents routinely kept their children at home, Down syndrome associations were flourishing, children with Down syndrome had been educated in public schools for years, books and articles celebrated the lives of children with Down syndrome, and *Life Goes On* was a wildly popular TV drama. To assert, in this context, that all "Down children" were ruining families, or that most adults ended up in public institutions, was like asserting that there were gravity-free areas of the Midwest, where you could let go of a brick and watch it float up towards the clouds. The only difference is that a brick has no feelings, no aspirations, no wishes that can be stunted by authoritative lies.

p. 161   ***Stereotypes of character are presented as biological fact:*** The science writer Matt Ridley, in *Genome: The Autobiography of a*

Species in 23 Chapters (2006), writes: "Children born with an extra chromosome 21 are healthy, conspicuously happy, and destined to live for many years. But they are not considered, in that pejorative word, 'normal'. They have Down syndrome. Their characteristic appearance—short stature, plump bodies, narrow eyes, happy faces—is immediately familiar. So is the fact that they are mentally retarded, gentle and destined to age rapidly, often developing a form of Alzheimer's disease, and die before they reach the age of forty" (286–87).

This is not a description of Down syndrome. It is the Pillsbury Dough Boy, with an epicanthal fold. It is a mixture of fact, stereotype, and rumor, affirmed as genetic destiny. People with Down syndrome are not "destined" to die by a certain age; some die very early, and some live into their sixties. Variation in the population and the sharp rise in life expectancy make nonsense of any preset "destiny." (As of the second edition of Ridley's book, however, the life expectancy was about fifty-five.) Though people with Down syndrome are subject to higher rates of early-onset Alzheimer's, they do not "age rapidly." "Plumpness" is common but not inevitable; it is more likely, but then it is going to be more likely if your muscle tone tends to be worse, you are socially isolated, and you lack for recreational opportunities. (Indeed, these same problems contribute to high rates of depression in adults with Down syndrome. Presumably they are depressed, but in a plump, happy way.)

For other examples, see the note on "sweet," above.

p. 162   **the word "Mongol," and all its variants:** See, for example, the 1977 *Principles of Genetics*, by Irwin H. Herskowitz:

> *Down's syndrome (Mongolism)* in human beings is usually the result of trisomy for chromosome 21 (Figure 13-3). Affected individuals, who usually have a happy dis-

position, are handicapped by severe mental and physical retardation. They are characteristically obese and have a thick tongue, sagging mouth, unusual palm and sole prints, and an eyelid fold similar to that of members of the Mongoloid race. (326)

Healthy Healing: A Guide to Self-Healing for Everyone (11th ed., Traditional Wisdom, Inc., 2001) concludes a laundry list of "common symptoms" by claiming that "gland and hormone deficiencies [give] the person a 'retarded,' mongoloid appearance" (372). *Healthy Healing* also offers a startling list of "Common Causes" for Down syndrome, including "excess water fluoridation; too much sugar and refined foods; heavy metal poisoning altering brain chemistry; hypoglycemia and glycogen storage deficiency; allergies; birth trauma" (372).

p. 162   **"primates":** Monroe W. Strickberger's *Genetics* (New York: Macmillan, 1985) asserts that Down syndrome "is probably the most common congenital abnormality, with a frequence of one out of 600 births. It is characterized by mental retardation, a short body with stubby fingers, swollen tongue, monkey-like skin ridges on the extremities, and eyelid folds resembling those of Mongolian races" (423). (A footnote: "The same defect can be found in other primates, e.g. a young chimpanzee showing a large number of traits similar to those shown by human children with Down syndrome was also reported to be trisomic for one of the small acrocentric chromosomes in the G group (21?)" [423].)

p. 162   **The best make the developing individual central, not a footnote:** The British pediatrician Cliff Cunningham, in *Understanding Down's Syndrome: An Introduction for Parents*, frames his list with a reassuring warning: "This chapter emphasises the many characteristics and medical problems that have been associated with the condition. The majority of children with Down's syndrome will have only a small number of these characteristics, and will not be afflicted by all, if any, of the medical problems. Therefore please take care in relating the information to your baby or child" (86).

TRAGEDY AND EXPECTATION

p. 169   ***the child's arrival is a tragedy:*** It hardly seems necessary to cite the common belief that Down syndrome is a tragedy, but the connection is commented on by Barbara Katz Rothman, in *Genetic Maps and Human Imaginations*: "That is the story of prenatal diagnosis and selective abortion: genetic testing developed to prevent the births of babies whose lives were believed to be tragedies best avoided. The first such category diagnosed was fetuses with Down syndrome, but other disabilities were also understood to make life not worth living. . . . The birth of a disabled child was understood to be an unqualified tragedy from which women should be spared." See also Shapiro, *No Pity: People with Disabilities Forging a Civil Rights Movement*, 327.

p. 169   ***"a description of Down syndrome segues into predicted ruin":*** Snustad and Simmons, *Principles of Genetics*, 22.

p. 170   ***But Michael and Carole do not react in believable ways:*** For a real-life contrast, it's worth looking at a personal account ("Unexpected Outcomes—a Birth Story") published in the *International Journal of Childbirth Education* 15, no. 3 (2000). In it, Marcia Flinkstrom, a doula and childbirth educator, describes the birth of her seventh child, Kayla Nicole. The birth was normal. But as she looked at her child, Flinkstrom writes, "my heart began to sink." She continues: "A large knot began to form in my stomach and a mild sense of panic was growing. Something was not right. Her tongue seemed a bit too large for her mouth and she kept thrusting it outward" (12). A nurse agrees that the child might have Down syndrome, but Flinkstrom has to wait till the next morning, alone, to see a doctor.

> All night I stared and stared at my baby's face. I saw it, and I didn't. I felt okay, and minutes later I felt panic. The tears seemed to never end. . . . I wanted to go home and not necessarily take this baby with me. She didn't even have a name. The pit in my stomach grew larger and I was alone with this baby. She wasn't interested in nursing. Her tongue kept getting in the way. It was truly a dark night. (12)

But Flinkstrom's story, unlike Michael and Carole's, continues beyond the birth.

> The whole family grieved and tears flowed. Each child reacted in his or her own way. Friends were very supportive, listening to me over and over, holding me while I cried. A family gathering at the hospital two days after her birth brought the first bit of healing. With a birthday cake sporting a big "0" candle, we had a family vote to name our baby and celebrate her presence. Kayla Nicole was sung to and amidst the tears, I found some peace. The test results arrived two weeks later and confirmed our suspicions. The process of acceptance and healing would continue. (12)

Flinkstrom writes that as a childbirth educator, she is a better teacher for her own experience as a mother. But then, this is a common pattern in parental accounts. The story only looks like tragedy at first; in the long run, it turns out to be something else.

p. 173 *A normal child:* In a recent review article ("Families of Children with Down Syndrome: What We Know and What We Need to Know"), Monica Cuskelly, Penny Hauser-Cram, and Marcia van Riper describe a complex picture, something more like "increased difficulty" than outright tragedy. While acknowledging that many researchers found "lower levels of well-being" in families of children with Down syndrome, Cuskelly et al. also report a range of positive outcomes; van Riper herself found "similar levels of well-being to those experienced by parents of typically developing children," and benefits were also reported for siblings.

The authors also report that the belief that Down syndrome is a "tragedy" may itself be a factor in the family's experience. Other factors include community support (or lack thereof), the family's "belief systems," the presence of Early Intervention, the family's income, the child's age, and so on. Cuskelly et al. report that much work remains to be done in the field (including "the need for . . . a more balanced perspective—one that acknowledges both positive and negative aspects of the experience"). But the belief that a child with Down syndrome automatically leads to tragedy does not seem to be supported by current research.

p. 174 *a sensitive, informed, unbiased genetic counselor:* For a portrait of such a counselor, and for an in-depth look at a couple facing a positively diagnosed fetus, see Mitchell Zuckoff's *Choosing Naia: A Family's Journey* (Boston: Beacon Press, 2003).

p. 174 *Such an approach . . . will increase choice:* in Asch, "Prenatal Diagnosis and Selective Abortion," 1655.

JOHN LANGDON DOWN

Details about John Langdon Down's life and work at Earlswood asylum are drawn from O. Conor Ward's biography, and from David Wright's history of the asylum. Quotations from Down's writings are drawn from the collection *On Some of the Mental Affections of Childhood and Youth*, which includes his paper "Observations on an Ethnic Classification of Idiots."

p. 183   ***"In a remote part of the country":*** quoted in Ward, *John Langdon Down, 1828–1896: A Caring Pioneer*, 7.

p. 184   ***According to his biographer:*** Down's pharmaceutical innovations are reported in Ward, *Caring Pioneer*, 11; his attitude towards the shop, in a letter to his brother-in-law, are quoted in Ward, 15.

p. 184   ***In 1853 . . . he left to become a doctor:*** He had been preparing to leave for some time: though his goal was to attend medical school, he had seriously considered a research career in chemistry, and had even learned German, in order to work with a particular professor abroad. Learning a new language for your *backup* choice does not suggest a young man who intended to stick around.

p. 184   ***there are two public versions of Down:*** Wright, *Mental Disability in Victorian England*, 155.

p. 185   ***his patients, whom he referred to as "family members":*** Collins, *Not Even Wrong*, 133.

p. 185   ***"difficult to realise . . . difficult to believe":*** Down, "Observations," 214, 213.

p. 186   *as much variation* within *the entire continent of Africa:* Marks, *What It Means to Be 98% Chimpanzee*, 83–84.

p. 187   *as several writers have pointed out:* For example, see Wright, *Mental Disability in Victorian England*, 165; and Gould, "Dr. Down's Syndrome," 166.

p. 187   *"Here, however, we have examples of retrogression":* Down, *Mental Affections*, 216.

p. 195   *"The tendency in science":* Stepan, *Idea of Race in Science*, xviii.

In my view, Down did not absorb the history of racial science, then translate it into theory. Instead, he likely appropriated the words of an earlier theorist of race: Johann Friedrich von Blumenbach. According to Ward, Down's theory was triggered by reading Thomas Bendyshe's 1865 translation of Blumenbach's *On the Natural Variety of Humankind*. When I finally looked up the translation, I found a startling similarity between Down's descriptions of his racialized "idiots," and Blumenbach's descriptions of race, as the following examples attest.

Blumenbach, on "Ethiopians":

.. malar bones protruding outwards; eyes very prominent . . . the lips (especially the upper) very puffy; chin retreating. (266)

Down, on "several well-marked examples of the Ethiopian variety":

[They present] the characteristic malar bones, the prominent eyes, the puffy lips, and retreating chin. (212)

Blumenbach, on the "Malay variety":

> ... hair black, soft, curly, thick and plentiful ... mouth large, upper jaw somewhat prominent with the parts of the face when seen in profile. .... This last variety includes the islanders of the Pacific Ocean. (266)

Down, writing that "some arrange themselves around the Malay variety":

> [They] present in their soft, black, curly hair, their prominent upper jaws and capacious mouths, types of the family which people the South Sea Islands. (213)

Blumenbach, on "the American variety":

> ... forehead short; eyes set very deep; nose somewhat apish, but prominent. (266)

Down:

> Nor has there been wanting the analogues of the people who with shortened foreheads, prominent cheeks, deep-set eyes, and slightly apish nose, originally inhabited the American Continent. (213)

Here is Blumenbach's description of "the countenance common to the Mongolian nations":

> Face wide, at the same time flat and depressed; the parts, therefore, indistinct and running into one another. Interspace between the eyes, or glabella, smooth, very wide. Nose flattened. Cheeks usually rounded, projecting outwards. Opening of the eyelids narrow, linear (*yeux bridès*). Chin, somewhat prominent. (228)

Here is Down's description of his "specimen" of Mongolian idiocy:

> The face is flat and broad, and destitute of prominence. The cheeks are roundish, and extended later-

ally. The eyes are obliquely placed, and the internal canthi more than normally distant from one another. The palpebral fissure is very narrow. (214)

Blumenbach describes Mongolian skin as having "a yellow, olive-tinge" (209); Down notes, "The skin has a slight dirty-yellowish tinge" (214). But it is Down's description of hair that most clearly illustrates the way he used his source. Here is Blumenbach, describing the hair first of Caucasians, then of Mongolians:

> 1. The first of a brownish or nutty colour (*cendré*), shading off on the one side into yellow, on the other into black: soft, long, and undulating. Common in the nations of temperate Europe; formerly particularly famous among the inhabitants of ancient Germany.
>
> 2. The second, black, stiff, straight, and scanty; such as is common to the Mongolian and American nations. (224)

Down, trying to describe someone who was neither white nor Mongolian, but somehow both, averages the two descriptions:

> The hair is not black, as in the real Mongol, but of a brownish colour, straight and scanty. (214)

In the conclusion of his "Observations," Down, as we have seen, resolves his racial views with paradox. It is an odd, startling move:

> I cannot but think that the observations which I have recorded are indications that the difference in the races are not specific, but variable. These examples of the result of degeneracy among mankind appear to me to furnish some argument in favour of the unity of the human species. (216–17)

This passage is often cited as proof of Down's liberal views on race. That's true, as far as it goes. But it also illustrates his approach to other thinkers, because this is Blumenbach's conclusion too. At the end of his treatise, after rehearsing his argument about "the causes and ways of degeneration," Blumenbach asserts, in italics,

> That no doubt can any longer remain but that we are with great probability right in referring all and singular as many varieties of man as are at present known to one and the same species. (276)

Down, in other words, was a peculiarly modern writer, a collagist, a writer of pastiche. It also seems likely that all of his ethnic idiots, except for the "Mongolian," were invented to fill out his system. (Although Down's photographs of people with Down syndrome survive, there are no credible instances of any other ethnic type.)

p. 196 *a scientist and a family man:* in Wolstenholme and Porter, *Mongolism*, 1–5.

p. 197 *the discussion that follows:* in Wolstenholme and Porter, *Mongolism*, 88–90.

One should not assume too much about the writers, based on their use of the word "Mongol." Lionel Penrose, for instance, was the leading expert on Down syndrome at the time, and had written a foreword to the first autobiography of a person with Down syndrome: *The World of Nigel Hunt: The Diary of a Mongoloid Youth* (New York: Garrett Publications, 1967), by Nigel Hunt, published that same year. Douglas Hunt, Nigel's father, also uses the word "mongoloid."

p. 197   *a photograph of a family member unmentioned:* Ward, *Caring Pioneer,* 142.

ENGINEERING

p. 205   *"the problem of bereavement":* Wilmut and Highfield, *After Dolly,* 131.

p. 206   *a description. . . . that splices science with longing:* Wilmut and Highfield, *After Dolly,* 162.

p. 206   ***Beside other projections of our genetic future:*** As far as Ian Wilmut is concerned, Lee Silver's scenarios "have no bearing upon reality" (Wilmut and Highfield, *After Dolly,* 266). He also notes that even as Dolly was in utero, "the Princeton professor Lee Silver was writing a popular book . . . in which he was patiently explaining why cloning from adults was a biological impossibility" (124).

p. 207   *"the lung-modified thick-skinned dark green descendants":* Silver, *Remaking Eden,* 289.

p. 207   ***artificial chromosomes containing "gene-packs":*** Silver, *Remaking Eden,* 271.

p. 208   ***a technical problem:*** Wilmut and Highfield, *After Dolly,* 214 and 255–56; Silver, *Remaking Eden,* 121. Wilmut's perspective and Silver's are hardly identical: Wilmut writes, for example, "I believe that we ought to accept ourselves and our children for what we are, rather than attempting to breed an improved race of human beings" (266)—a sentiment alien to Silver's book. However, Wilmut also concludes one chapter with the hope of "eradicating human genetic diseases" (222), of which Down syndrome, for him at least, is clearly one.

p. 211 ***Our jokes . . . are all diagnoses:*** See, for example, Michael Bérubé's *Life as We Know It*: "Right through the 1970s, "mongoloid idiot" wasn't an epithet; it was a *diagnosis*" (27). See also the disability activist Kathie Snow's article "The Hierarchy of Insults": "Listen to talk radio, watch a sitcom, or just pay attention to your own conversations at home or work, and you'll hear 'retard,' 'idiot,' 'moron,' 'imbecile,' 'lame,' 'crazy,' 'schizo,' 'spaz,' and more. . . . What these and other words have in common is that they were, or are, *medical diagnoses*" (accessed at http://www.disabilityisnatural.com/images/PDF/hierinsults.pdf).

p. 211 ***as with anabolic steroids:*** McKibben, *Enough*, 62–63.

p. 212 ***the improved are destined to be inferior:*** The consequence of continual upgrades, for McKibben, is a loss of connection with preceding generations, who are unenhanced, and with following generations, who are *more* enhanced. Not only will the hypothetical child "glance back over his shoulder and see a gap between himself and human history," he will also be unable to imagine connection with future children, who are "Windows 2050 to his Atari." McKibben, *Enough*, 64–65.

p. 212 ***"into the ultraviolet range":*** Silver, *Remaking Eden*, 279.

Bibliography

Asch, Adrienne. "Prenatal Diagnosis and Selective Abortion: A Challenge to Practice and Policy." *American Journal of Public Health* 89, no. 11 (1999): 1649–56.

Beck, Martha Nibley. *Expecting Adam*. New York: Berkley Books, 2000.

Benda, Clemens. *Mongolism and Cretinism: A Study of the Clinical Manifestations and the General Pathology of Pituitary and Thyroid Deficiency*. New York: Grune & Stratton, 1946.

Bérubé, Michael. *Life as We Know It: A Father, a Family, and an Exceptional Child*. New York: Pantheon Books, 1996.

Blumenbach, Johann Friedrich. *The Anthropological Treatises of Johann Friedrich Blumenbach*. Translated by Thomas Bendyshe. London: Published for the Anthropological Society by Longman, Green, Longman, Roberts, and Green. 1865.

Brousseau, Kate. *Mongolism: A Study of the Physical and Mental Characteristics of Mongolian Imbeciles*. Baltimore: Williams and Wilkins Company, 1928.

Buffon, Georges-Louis Leclerc, Comte de. *Natural History, General and Particular*. Translated by William Smellie. London: T. Cadell and W. Davies, 1812.

Collins, Paul. *Not Even Wrong: A Father's Journey into the Lost History of Autism*. New York: Bloomsbury, 2004.

Crosby, Anne. *Matthew: A Son's Life, a Mother's Story*. Philadelphia: Paul Dry Books, 2006.

Cunningham, Cliff. *Understanding Down Syndrome: An Introduction for Parents*. Cambridge, MA: Brookline Books, 1988.

Cuskelly, Monica, Penny Hauser-Cram, and Marcia Van Riper. "Families of Children with Down Syndrome: What We Know and What We Need to Know." *Down Syndrome Research and Practice*. Advance online publication, July 4, 2008. Accessed at http://www.down-syndrome.org/reviews/2079/reviews-2079.pdf.

Down, John Langdon. *On Some of the Mental Affections of Childhood and Youth*. London: J. A. Churchill, 1887.

Estreich, Ranko. "Remembering How Things Were." Typescript.

Gould, Stephen Jay. "Dr. Down's Syndrome." In *The Panda's Thumb: More Reflections in Natural History*. 1980, reprint; London: Penguin, 1990.

Griffiths, Anthony, Jeffrey H. Miller, David T. Suzuki, Richard C. Lewontin, and William M. Gelbart, eds. *Introduction to Genetic Analysis*. New York: W. H. Freeman, 1996.

Herskowitz, Irwin H. *Principles of Genetics*. New York: Macmillan, 1977.

Kingsley, Emily Perl. "Welcome to Holland." In *You Will Dream New Dreams: Inspiring Personal Stories by Parents of Children with Disabilities*. Edited by Stanley D. Klein and Kim Schive, 216–17. New York: Kensington, 2001.

Marks, Jonathan. *What It Means to Be 98% Chimpanzee: Apes, People, and Their Genes*. Berkeley: University of California Press, 2002.

McKibben, Bill. *Enough: Staying Human in an Engineered Age*. New York: Henry Holt and Company, 2003.

Milunsky, Aubrey. *Your Genetic Destiny: Know Your Genes, Secure Your Health, Save Your Life*. Cambridge, MA: Perseus, 2001.

Murkoff, Heidi Eisenberg, Arlene Eisenberg, and Sandee Eisenberg Hathaway. *What to Expect the First Year*. New York: Workman, 2003.

Ridley, Matt. *Genome: The Autobiography of a Species in 23 Chapters.* New York: HarperPerennial, 2006.

Rothman, Barbara Katz. *Genetic Maps and Human Imaginations: The Limits of Science in Understanding Who We Are.* New York: W. W. Norton, 1998.

Selikowitz, Mark. *Down Syndrome: The Facts.* Oxford: Oxford University Press, 1997.

Shapiro, Joseph. *No Pity: People with Disabilities Forging a Civil Rights Movement.* New York: Times Books, 1993.

Shelov, Steven P., editor-in-chief; Tanya Remer Altmann, associate medical editor; Robert E. Hannemann, associate medical editor, emeritus; and Richard Trubo. *Caring for Your Baby and Young Child: Birth to Age 5.* New York: Bantam Books, 2009.

Silver, Lee. *Remaking Eden: How Genetic Engineering and Cloning Will Transform the American Family.* New York: HarperPerennial, 2007.

Skotko, Brian. "Mothers of Children with Down Syndrome Reflect on Their Postnatal Support." *Pediatrics* 115, no. 1 (2005): 64–77.

Sloan, Kathy. *To Mend a Broken Heart.* Atlanta: Pritchett & Hull, 1998.

Snustad, D. Peter, and Michael J. Simmons. *Principles of Genetics.* 3rd ed. Hoboken, NJ: John Wiley and Sons, 2003.

Stepan, Nancy. *The Idea of Race in Science: Great Britain, 1800–1960.* London: Macmillan, 1982.

Stout, Lucille. *I Reclaimed My Child: The Story of a Family into Which a Retarded Child Was Born.* Philadelphia: Chilton, 1959.

Stray-Gundersen, Karen. *Babies with Down Syndrome: A New Parents' Guide.* 2nd ed. Woodbine House, 1995.

Trainer, Marilyn. *Differences in Common: Straight Talk on Mental Retardation, Down Syndrome, and Life.* Bethesda, MD: Woodbine House, 1991.

Van Dyke, Don C., Philip Mattheis, Susan Eberly, and Janet Williams, eds. *Medical and Surgical Care for Children with Down Syndrome: A Guide for Parents.* Bethesda, MD: Woodbine House, 1995.

Ward, O. Conor. *John Langdon Down, 1828–1896: A Caring Pioneer.* London: Royal Society of Medicine Press, 1998.

Wegman, William. *One, Two, Three.* New York: Hyperion, 1995.

Wilmut, Ian, and Roger Highfield. *After Dolly: The Uses and Misuses of Human Cloning.* New York: Norton, 2006.

Wolstenholme, G. E. W., and Ruth Porter, eds. *Mongolism: In Commemoration of Dr. John Langdon Haydon Down.* London: Churchill, 1967.

Wright, David. *Mental Disability in Victorian England: The Earlswood Asylum, 1847–1901.* Oxford: Oxford University Press, 2001.

Zuckoff, Mitchell. *Choosing Naia: A Family's Journey.* Boston: Beacon, 2003.

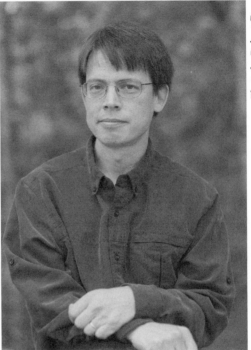
Photo by Robert Don

George Estreich's collection of poems, *Textbook Illustrations of the Human Body,* won the Gorsline Prize and was published in 2004 by Cloudbank Books. He lives in Corvallis, Oregon, with his wife Theresa, a research scientist, and his two daughters, Ellie and Laura.